New Roles for Psychiatrists in Organized Systems of Care

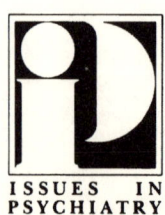

Joseph D. Bloom, M.D.
Series Editor

New Roles for Psychiatrists in Organized Systems of Care

Edited by

Jeremy A. Lazarus, M.D.
and
Steven S. Sharfstein, M.D.

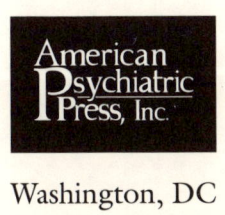

Washington, DC
London, England

Note: The authors have worked to ensure that all information in this book concerning drug dosages, schedules, and routes of administration is accurate as of the time of publication and consistent with standards set by the U.S. Food and Drug Administration and the general medical community. As medical research and practice advance, however, therapeutic standards may change. For this reason and because human and mechanical errors sometimes occur, we recommend that readers follow the advice of a physician who is directly involved in their care or the care of a member of their family.

Books published by the American Psychiatric Press, Inc., represent the views and opinions of the individual authors and do not necessarily represent the policies and opinions of the Press or the American Psychiatric Association.

Copyright © 1998 American Psychiatric Press, Inc.
ALL RIGHTS RESERVED
Manufactured in the United States of America on acid-free paper
First Edition
01 00 99 98   4 3 2 1

American Psychiatric Press, Inc.
1400 K Street, N.W.
Washington, DC 20005
www.appi.org

Library of Congress Cataloging-in-Publication Data
New roles for psychiatrists in organized systems of care / edited by
  Jeremy A. Lazarus and Steven S. Sharfstein. — 1st ed.
     p.   cm.
  Includes bibliographical references and index.
  ISBN 0-88048-758-5 (alk. paper)
  1. Psychiatry—Practice—United States.   2. Managed mental health care—United States.   I. Lazarus, Jeremy A.   II. Sharfstein, Steven S. (Steven Samuel), 1942– .
  [DNLM: 1. Psychiatry—trends. 2. Managed Care Programs—trends. WM 21 N532 1998]
  RC465.5.N49   1998
  362.2—dc21
  DNLM/DC
  For Library of Congress   97-50111
                                                                                         CIP

British Library Cataloguing-in-Publication Data
A CIP record is available from the British Library.

Contents

Contributors ix

Introduction xi
  Jeremy A. Lazarus, M.D., and Steven S. Sharfstein, M.D.

Section I: The Transformation of American Psychiatry by Managed Care

CHAPTER ONE

The Emergence of Organized Systems of Care 3
  Anne M. Stoline, M.D.

CHAPTER TWO

Quality in Managed Care Systems:
What Is in the Patient's Best Interests? 23
  Alex R. Rodriguez, M.D.

Section II: Roles for Psychiatrists in the New Medical Marketplace

CHAPTER THREE

Psychiatrists and the New Managed Systems of Care:
Roles and Responsibilities 41
  Lloyd I. Sederer, M.D.

CHAPTER FOUR

Clinical Role of the Psychiatrist in Managed Care 57
Alan A. Axelson, M.D.

CHAPTER FIVE

Administrative Psychiatry and Managed Care:
Advances and Opportunities 71
Ronald D. Geraty, M.D.

CHAPTER SIX

The Future of Private Office Practice of Psychiatry in an
Environment Dominated by Managed Care 87
Norman A. Clemens, M.D.

Section III: Training, Guidelines, and Ethics

CHAPTER SEVEN

Psychiatric Training and Managed Care 111
James E. Sabin, M.D.

CHAPTER EIGHT

Practice Guidelines and Outcomes Management:
Future Roles for Psychiatrists 123
John C. Bartlett, M.D., M.P.H.

CHAPTER NINE

The Physician-Patient Relationship in a Managed Care Setting:
Informed Consent, Confidentiality, and Trust 141
Elaine M. Buzzinotti, J.D., Loren H. Roth, M.D., M.P.H., and Thomas L. Horn, M.D.

CHAPTER TEN

New Financial Incentives and
Disincentives in Psychiatry 169
Jeremy A. Lazarus, M.D.

Section IV: The Future for Psychiatry in Organized Systems of Care

CHAPTER ELEVEN

Paradigms, Preemptions, and Stages:
Understanding the Transformation of
American Psychiatry by Managed Care 187
Alan A. Stone, M.D.

CHAPTER TWELVE

The Identity of the Field in the Context of
Changing Roles 239
John J. Boronow, M.D., and Steven S. Sharfstein, M.D.

Index 261

Contributors

Alan A. Axelson, M.D.
President and Medical Director, InterCare Psych Services, Pittsburgh, Pennsylvania

John C. Bartlett, M.D., M.P.H.
Atlanta, Georgia

John J. Boronow, M.D.
Senior Psychiatrist, Sheppard and Enoch Pratt Hospital, Towson, Maryland

Elaine M. Buzzinotti, J.D.
Assistant Counsel and Associate Administrator, Western Psychiatric Institute and Clinic of the University of Pittsburgh Medical Center, Pittsburgh, Pennsylvania

Norman A. Clemens, M.D.
Clinical Professor of Psychiatry, Case Western Reserve University, Cleveland, Ohio

Ronald D. Geraty, M.D.
President, Continuum Behavioral Healthcare Corporation, Park Ridge, New Jersey

Thomas L. Horn, M.D.
Assistant Professor of Psychiatry, University of Pittsburgh School of Medicine; Chief of Clinical Services, Western Psychiatric Institute and Clinic of the University of Pittsburgh Medical Center, Pittsburgh, Pennsylvania

Jeremy A. Lazarus, M.D.
Associate Clinical Professor of Psychiatry, University of Colorado Health Sciences Center, Denver, Colorado

Alex R. Rodriguez, M.D.
Vice President and Medical Director, Consortium Health Plans, Inc., Columbia, Maryland; Lecturer in Psychiatry, Yale University School of Medicine, New Haven, Connecticut

Loren H. Roth, M.D., M.P.H.
Professor and Vice Chairman of Psychiatry, Associate Vice Chancellor for Education for Health Sciences, University of Pittsburgh Medical Center, Pittsburgh, Pennsylvania

James E. Sabin, M.D.
Associate Clinical Professor of Psychiatry, Harvard Medical School, Cambridge, Massachussetts; Co-Director, Center for Ethics in Managed Care, Harvard Pilgrim Health Care and Harvard Medical School, Cambridge, Massachussetts

Lloyd I. Sederer, M.D.
Senior Vice President, Clinical Services, McLean Hospital, Belmont, Massachussetts; Associate Professor of Clinical Psychiatry, Harvard Medical School, Cambridge, Massachussetts

Steven S. Sharfstein, M.D.
President, Medical Director, CEO, Sheppard Pratt Health System, Inc.; Clinical Professor of Psychiatry, University of Maryland

Anne M. Stoline, M.D.
Director, Women's Mental Health, Mercy Medical Center, Baltimore, Maryland

Alan A. Stone, M.D.
Touroff-Gluéck Professor of Law and Psychiatry, Faculty of Law and Faculty of Medicine, Harvard University Law School, Cambridge, Massachussetts

Introduction

Jeremy A. Lazarus, M.D., and Steven S. Sharfstein, M.D.

The practice of medicine in America is being transformed by the new medical marketplace. Managed care has changed opportunities for access to quality services and has rewritten the financial incentives for physicians. This impact has been keenly felt in the medical specialty of psychiatry.

Psychiatry, perhaps more than any other medical specialty, provides diverse opportunities for work. Psychiatrists perform many productive roles in clinical medicine, including the care and treatment of patients with mental disorders in a variety of settings. These settings have included both hospital and nonhospital locations in the private and public sectors, in solo and group practices. Psychiatrists also fulfill a range of consultative, management, and leadership roles within health and human services. Due to the robust epidemiology of mental disorders and the social consequences of untreated mental illness, a strong demand for a psychiatrist's work exists. Psychiatrists are intimately involved in the functionings of our legal and educational systems and throughout the workplace as well. In all of these institutions and settings, psychiatrists must abide by their medical ethics, which include patient advocacy, confidentiality, honesty, and the maxim to "above all do no harm."

The transformation of American medicine and psychiatry is a rewriting of traditional autonomous private practice into a corporate organized system of care. As psychiatrists function in new managed systems of care, what is the impact on our traditional ethics and on the quality of the care provided to patients? How should psychiatrists lead rather than follow this revolution in the financing of health care delivery? Can psychiatrists adapt and survive as a medical specialty in the face of the severe challenge to our traditional and time-honored healing role?

This book and the conference that inspired it is an effort to address these questions in a forthright manner, posing the tough questions, analyzing the necessity for a creative, ethically informed response to this revolutionary revision in the financing of health care.

Many psychiatrists these days find themselves uncertain and anxious about their future. Observing this anxiety, medical students select medical specialties other than psychiatry, especially primary care. Psychiatrists who do not appreciate the power of the new medical marketplace find themselves out in the cold if they have not joined networks, health maintenance organizations, or other corporatized forms of referral and care delivery. This book is intended to help psychiatrists understand this transformation and to proactively anticipate the essential role they need to play in returning the control of care to the doctor/patient relationship.

This book is organized into four parts. The first part sets the stage for the broad social trends and forces of medical economics that have transformed the profession. The two chapters by Drs. Stoline and Rodriguez provide a broad overview of the issues that have brought us to managed care. With a sense of the history and purposes of our field and the role psychiatrists can play in managed care delivery systems, they introduce the chapters that follow.

The second section more explicitly and directly describes the functions for psychiatrists in the newly emerging organizations of care. The chapters by Drs. Sederer, Axelson, Geraty, and Clemens provide different perspectives on these roles, including the relationship of psychiatrists to other mental health professionals and primary care practitioners, the continuing need for and compelling logic of private practice, and new administrative positions for psychiatrists in organized care systems.

The third section of the book focuses on training, practice guidelines, and explicit discussions of the changed physician/patient relationship. Ms. Buzzinotti and Drs. Sabin, Bartlett, Roth, and Horn focus on these closely associated issues as we approach the twenty-first century. Ethical concerns about the new financial incentives that challenge the traditional ethics of medicine are raised by Dr. Lazarus in the final chapter of this section.

The final section has two concluding chapters that shape a future vision for the profession. Dr. Stone prognosticates on the outcome of market forces on psychiatry and, by derivation, the rest of medicine. The final chapter by Drs. Boronow and Sharfstein further predicts the changes in the identity of the field in the context of modified roles.

This book emerges from a conference that took place in Raleigh-Durham, North Carolina, in October 1994. Recognizing the crisis and challenge at hand, the American Psychiatric Association, through its Managed Care and Ethics Committees, put together the conference, which brought together APA leaders, medical directors of managed care companies, clinicians, and legal and ethical experts in an intensive, two-day dialogue on topics of great interest to the field. This conference was the second of two, the first—on ethics and managed care—having taken place two years earlier at Sheppard Pratt. That conference, whose proceedings have been published (American Psychiatric Association), began the exchange on these subjects between the leaders of American psychiatry and the newly emerging managed care industry.

The editors are especially grateful to the Boroughs Wellcome Company, which supported both conferences. We would like to give special thanks to Carol Davis, Emma Wilkens, George Campbell, Sajini Thomas, Jim Larson, Katherine Chambless, Ruth Yoshpe, and Christine Lehmann at the APA, who provided the essential support for these conferences.

As the new medical marketplace downsizes the health care industry in an effort to contain costs, we, as physicians and leaders in our field, must fully understand the impact of these modifications in the doctor/patient relationship. We hope this book will stimulate further discussion, research, and a better appreciation of the changes taking place.

Reference

American Psychiatric Association: Transcript Summary from the Ethics in Managed Care Conference. Sheppard Pratt Hospital, Baltimore, Maryland, October 25–26, 1991

Section I
The Transformation of American Psychiatry by Managed Care

CHAPTER ONE

The Emergence of Organized Systems of Care

Anne M. Stoline, M.D.

Only 200 years ago, psychiatrists had very little understanding of the causes of psychiatric symptoms. Their limited treatments, including exorcism and bloodletting, were harsh and ineffective. Public funds provided the barest resources for the warehousing of patients in jails and later in spartan asylums. As a result, patients with major mental illness were condemned to suffer with chronic symptoms and impaired functioning.

Today we know much more about the pathophysiology of mental illnesses and have a vast armamentarium of pharmacologic and psychotherapeutic tools at our disposal. Yet because recent reforms in public and private health care funding have severely constrained the resources available to the mental health sector, many psychiatrists feel they lack adequate tools to provide care, creating a situation akin to that of our predecessors. Despite two centuries of scientific progress and the development of numerous effective psychiatric treatments, we wonder whether the mentally ill suffer unnecessarily as a result of cost-cutting policy choices. Why are resources so limited when our ability to aid those with psychiatric impairment has grown so substantially? The reason for this paradox lies in social attitudes, economic trends, and political decisions that affect health care resource allocation; clinical and scientific progress are not independent factors in the evolution of the health care system. One major response to changes in funding and health policy was the emergence of organized systems of care. In this chapter we will examine recent history to shed light on the forces influencing their growth and development.

Three distinct eras may be discerned in the last four decades of United States health care policy. The first was brought about by a crisis in access to health care by the elderly and the indigent in the 1960s. Associated with the reform movement that arose in response to this crisis was the effort to move as many patients as possible out of psychiatric institutions and to mainstream them within society. The second era, beginning in the 1970s, was characterized by steep inflation in health care costs. Those paying for care—government, private employers, and insurers—implemented cost control measures that caused fundamental changes in United States health care delivery. The third era, the most complex of the three, has seen the problems in medicine and psychiatry from the previous two eras compounded by a variety of new concerns, including the effects of stringent cost control and overregulation of medical care.

Social Forces Catalyze Reform in the 1960s

By the 1960s, it is possible to perceive the broad outlines of the health care system as we know it today—a heterogeneous collection of public and private systems more accurately termed a "nonsystem" because it developed without the influence of an overarching philosophy or vision. Mental health care in particular was divided into public and private sectors, a two-tiered and two-class arrangement made more distinct after creation of the private insurance industry in the 1930s.

The history of United States public sector psychiatry until the 1960s was synonymous with the history of its asylums, which provided care to indigent and chronically ill psychiatric patients. Although the private system benefited from the infusion of insurance dollars, the public system remained dependent on limited funds allocated by local, state, and federal government budgets. These large, predominantly rural, institutions had changed little in the previous 100 years. Conditions were austere at best.

As a result, the psychiatrist remained a poor stepchild to private sector colleagues despite the development of new psychiatric treatments and consequent expansion of the psychiatrist's role in the public sector. With only modest resources, the public sector psychiatrist was expected to care for a large population of chronically ill individuals. Even the revolution in psychiatric care brought about by the discovery of psychopharmacologic agents in the 1950s had not fundamentally changed public sector psychiatry. Although deinstitutionalization became clinically possible for many patients and the number of patients in asylums peaked in the mid-1950s, asylums were far from extinct, housing those with severe and persistent illness as well as longtime residents lacking social supports. Initially hailed as a positive step for asylum residents, deinstitutionalization left too many indigent and ill individuals homeless and without adequate outpatient support. In the early 1960s, harsh conditions within asylums and the plight of the homeless mentally ill became national issues in a social atmosphere growing ripe for reform.

Substantial problems existed for general medical care as well. By 1960, over 60% of the U.S. population was covered under some type of private insurance plan. The poor, however, did not benefit from the growth in private insurance coverage. The geriatric population was particularly at risk—50% of the elderly had no health insurance, and another 25% had inadequate coverage. While certain of payment from middle- and upper-class patients, most of whom were covered by insurance, many hospitals did not admit the poor or uninsured, transferring these patients to public facilities. Many impoverished families, particularly in rural areas, had no access to adequate care.

These problems were deemed intolerable by liberal social reformers in the 1960s, who spawned a movement that found favor during Kennedy's presidency, was carried over due to his legacy into the Johnson years, and was further supported by a prosperous economic era. With this coalescence of socioeconomic conditions favorable to reform, potential solutions to the access problem were debated at the national level. Health care was declared a citizen's right, and access to care became a popular political theme. Broad support developed for the use of public funds to provide medical care of the highest possible quality to the underprivileged in the population, resulting in the passage in 1965 of legislation creating the Medicare and Medicaid programs. Instituted in 1966, these plans offer coverage to the U.S. population over age 65 or to those meeting criteria for poverty or disability.

Medicare benefits are federally mandated, whereas states design their own Medicaid programs under broad federal guidelines. Both programs include inpatient and outpatient psychiatric care but exclude many of the community support and long-term services needed by people with severe and persistent mental illness. Outpatient benefits initially were quite limited under the Medicare program but were significantly increased in subsequent years. Provision of mental health coverage—however limited—for many patients otherwise unable to afford psychiatric care was a boon to the private mental health sector. Private sector hospital treatment was supported, although care in "institutions for mental disease" was intentionally limited in order to avoid federal responsibility for chronic care of the mentally ill. In fact, both Medicare and Medicaid benefits were designed to limit coverage to acute psychiatric treatment, leaving long-term treatment of the chronically ill in the hands of locally- and state-funded asylums.

The passage of Medicare and Medicaid legislation was a watershed in the history of government's role in the United States health care system. It followed nearly 30 years of debate about health care financing reform and effectively transferred primary responsibility for health care within the public sector from the local to the federal level. The extent of this federal financial commitment was unanticipated by legislators, and its budgetary consequences set the stage for further reform in the next decade.

In this wave of health care reform, Medicare and Medicaid legislation was preceded by passage of the Community Mental Health Center (CMHC) Act in 1963, which addressed the needs of those who were unable to afford private rates for outpatient care. The CMHC Act also reflected the beliefs that coordinated community-based services were the most appropriate way to deliver mental health care as well as provide a focus for prevention of mental illness. It encouraged the development of a network of outpatient, day treatment, and inpatient services and provided a structure to shift from the states to the federal government the costs of community services and outpatient care for patients released from asylums. The CMHC Act increased access to mental health services for many patients, particularly those in inner city and rural areas.

Attempting to diversify to outpatient services, the public sector was never adequately equipped to provide all services needed by those with mental illness. In many areas of the country, CMHCs overpromised their services, particularly with regard to delivery of community care to individuals with severe and persistent mental illness. In effect, the CMHC movement propelled the deinstitutionalization movement without providing adequate support services in local communities.

The CMHC Act affected the private sector as well. By expanding the public mental health sector from its previous role solely as a hospital system, it in effect relieved the private outpatient sector of responsibility for delivering care to uninsured, indigent patients. For these reasons, the act failed to solve the problem of inadequate mental health services available for those with severe mental illnesses (Foley and Sharfstein 1983).

The health policy reforms of the 1960s resulted in implementation of substantial and expensive programs that were nevertheless only partial solutions to the problems they were intended to correct. They did not provide comprehensive care, nor did they reach all needy individuals. Public asylums remained the provider of last resort.

Economic Forces Catalyze Reform in the 1970s

United States health care costs began to skyrocket in the 1960s, fueled by the growing private insurance industry as well as by the new federal mandates. A "health care cost crisis" was first described in the early 1970s. The reasons for severe cost increases are complex and numerous, but several factors predominate. General cost inflation during those years played a role, although health care costs consistently rose faster than general inflation. Population growth accounted for some of the increase. As medical care became ever more successful, the average life expectancy increased; the extension of life with the inevitable decline of health in late life due to chronic illnesses contributed to rising costs.

Continuous technological advances in medical care made available more clinical tests and treatments. Americans came to expect high-technology care, regardless of price, and became much more inclined to file lawsuits when outcomes were poor. Physicians responded to these pressures with risk-averse (and expensive) practice styles, resulting in steep increases in costs per case.

All of these factors contributed to rising costs, but perhaps the most inflationary aspect of the health care industry was the role played by health insurance. The private insurance industry was firmly established by this era, removing most of the financial consequences of medical decisions from patients and guaranteeing reimbursements to physicians. This arrangement created incentives for a "more is better" attitude by patients and physicians toward medical care. In those years, insurance companies simply paid the bills submitted to them, known as fee-for-service (FFS) reimbursement. This payment method does not reward cost-conscious decisions about resource use and consequently pushes costs higher. The Medicare and Medicaid programs exacerbated this aspect of the cost problem by increasing the pool of patients receiving care under more-is-better insurance incentives.

These general factors drove up mental health care costs as well. In addition, mental health care expenditures grew due to a sharp rise in the number of private, for-profit psychiatric facilities in the 1980s. Increased admissions to inpatient adult and adolescent units as well as a sharp rise in substance abuse treatment costs for both adults and juveniles also drove up expenditures (Frank, et al. 1991).

Because of the widespread use of private insurance coverage and public health care subsidies, by the 1970s and 1980s health care cost inflation affected the third-party payers of care—government, private insurers, and United States corporations—much more than it did most individuals.[1] The "cost crisis" evolved during these years as each of the major payers recognized health care costs as a problem.

Public policymakers were first to react to the cost problem; despite the intentions of policy architects in the 1960s to limit federal responsibility for medical expenditures, the federal government had since be-

---

[1] By 1990, health care costs were paid approximately 40% by government, with 60% from private sector sources. Only 20% derived from out-of-pocket payments by individuals. Due to their subsidies of employee health insurance, employers are estimated to have paid almost 30% of overall expenditures in 1990.

come the major payer of United States health care costs. But, whereas the federal financial commitment to health care was increasing, the 1960s also witnessed an economic slowdown that began and continued into the 1970s. Health care began to stand out as an area where savings could be made, particularly because analysts began to question whether these burgeoning expenditures were actually purchasing improved health. Some critics argued that the costs were not yielding the expected reductions in morbidity and mortality rates. As time went on, legislators grew less interested in health as a social issue and more interested in restraining health care costs. This change was complete by the 1970s, as politicians supported slowing the growth of the health care sector instead of offering carte blanche funds for its expansion.

Beginning in the 1970s, large employers first became concerned with escalating health care costs. Inflation in health care prices occurred at a time when United States productivity lagged behind that of other countries, and competition with foreign manufacturers was fierce. Many corporate executives realized the extent to which health care costs were reducing company profits. Whereas for decades, employers simply had paid the bill for employee health insurance premiums, widespread private sector concern with the cost problem was evident by the 1980s as employers reexamined their fringe benefit packages and began to implement health care spending restraints.

Insurance companies, too, joined the battle against the high costs of health care, although their expenditure increases could be (and were) passed along as higher premiums. Noting decreases in private insurance enrollment that reflected the conversion by many corporations to self-insurance programs, the disenrollment of individuals who could not afford steeply rising premiums, and the growth of alternative delivery systems such as health maintenance organizations (HMOs), insurance executives were motivated to implement their own cost containment measures.

Social attitudes played a role as well. The interests of "society" in containing health care costs vary according to one's definition of society. Taxpayers want to pay lower taxes; purchasers seek lower premiums; and patients want top-notch health care, which may not also be the least expensive or most efficient. These are all the same people, however, and their collective priorities shift over time. A survey in the early 1980s showed that cost control was a low priority, but as insurance premiums and medical expenses continued to rise and awareness of cost containment increased, opinions began to change. The public began to perceive rising health care costs as a problem. Although quality health care was valued, more and more Americans could not afford to obtain it. The news media drove this message home with references to the health care cost "crisis," and some 68% of those polled in a 1985 survey named cost as the greatest single problem facing the health care industry.

Cost Control Measures

Economic modeling of health care during the era of cost control created a new vocabulary in health policy that eventually became part of the vernacular. Applying classic market theory to medicine, health care became a *product* that is *supplied* by the health care sector (e.g., hospitals, other medical facilities, clinicians) and *demanded* by *consumers* (e.g., purchasers of insurance, policyholders, patients). *Demand-side* cost control methods attempt to influence patients' decisions, whereas *supply-side* methods target health care providers. (For a variety of reasons, health care is *not* a typical product, thus it should not be surprising that it has failed to respond to predictions and interventions based on traditional market models. These idiosyncrasies have not, however, dissuaded payers from implementing cost control strategies based on such theories.)

Many early cost containment efforts used demand-side strategies. Both public and private sector insurers increased cost sharing provisions, such as copayments and deductibles. In theory, these financial disincentives raise the threshold of severity for a patient to seek medical care. Preadmission certification, second surgical opinion requirements, gatekeeper programs, and numerous other oversight measures create analogous administrative disincentives.

Nixon's principal health policy effort was a demand-side strategy, the HMO Act of 1973, which intended to increase national enrollment in HMOs. Employers, too, created incentives for their employees to enroll in cost-saving capitated programs. National enrollment in HMOs did not increase significantly until the following decade, perhaps reflecting consumer resistance to stronger cost controls in the 1980s and ongoing availability of traditional plans.

Both financial and administrative demand-side strategies are ubiquitous today, although they are unable to reduce health care costs substantially. Although demand-side approaches heighten patients' awareness of their use of health care resources, their strongest effect is to delay the initial decision to seek care. Analysts attribute their failure to the fact that most subsequent resource use decisions are made by physicians.

Once payers realized that health care providers determine resource use (and hence expenditures), supply-side cost control measures became predominant. Early on, payers in both the public and private sectors implemented fee schedules and fee freezes on hospital and physician reimbursement. Although expenditures plateaued or declined (despite some providers who significantly increased their volume of services in order to maintain income), these measures did not incentivize cost-effective clinical behavior, thereby limiting their potential impact on health care cost increases.

Building on their experiences with these straightforward fee changes, private payers began to bargain with providers for reduced reimbursement rates. As agents for employers, insurers were encouraged to use aggressive tactics in negotiating fees and contracts. Particularly in urban areas, providers in some specialties feared dwindling patient volume if they declined these lower rates because demand-side administrative and financial incentives gave payers more control over patient flow. Today payers, not providers, generally set rates and contract terms.

In the public sector, the Resource-Based Relative Value System (RBRVS), implemented for Medicare reimbursement in 1992, targets physician reimbursement. The RBRVS sets an annual global annual budget from which physician Medicare payments are allocated. Physician groups exert substantial lobbying effort in order to influence the annual political process that updates the RBRVS fee schedule. Reimbursements are determined by service type, prior volumes, and weighted corrections intended to remedy long-standing disparities in payment to primary care and so-called cognitive services compared to subspecialty and surgical care, thereby controlling costs.

12 New Roles for Psychiatrists in Organized Systems of Care

None of the measures discussed to this point attempt to alter the traditional more-is-better economic incentive of fee-for-service (FFS) reimbursement. As the era of cost control continued, new financial incentives were introduced in the public and private sectors. For the first time, a substantial number of Americans began to receive care from providers receiving payment under less-is-more incentives. Although no payment measure is perfect, at least the weaknesses of the FFS payment method are familiar (i.e., its inflationary pressure and the risk that patients receive *more* services than are clinically indicated). The extent of the clinical and ethical consequences of the shift to less-is-more payment is not yet fully understood, nor are we at present a society comfortable with the implications of medicine practiced under these conditions.

The first federal reform that eliminated FFS financial incentives targeted hospitals because, as the most expensive site of care, they receive the bulk of Medicare payments. The Prospective Payment System (PPS) was implemented by the Medicare Program in 1983. The PPS is a hospital reimbursement system in which payment is prospectively determined, based primarily on a patient's diagnosis and procedures performed during hospitalization. Under PPS, cost-conscious resource use became necessary for institutional survival. No longer could a hospital be simply a workshop for practitioners. Hospital managers became actively involved in clinical medicine, monitoring physicians' practices for cost efficiency, encouraging use of preadmission testing, discouraging inpatient tests and procedures, and promoting rapid discharge. Under PPS, average hospital stays shortened, and the volume of ambulatory medical visits began to grow. Given the savings associated with reduced inpatient days, some analysts attribute the slowdown in health care cost increases in the 1980s to the effects of PPS.

Financial and administrative measures that directly influence physicians' clinical behavior are perhaps the most controversial cost control measures. With financial interventions including less-is-more reimbursement arrangements as well as capitated and prospectively based payments, some payers contracted to share financial risk with physicians. Administrative interventions that influence bedside decision making generally fall under the rubric of *managed care*. Broadly defined, managed care denotes a wide range of review and service delivery systems designed to control health care costs by controlling utilization of health care resources.

In the ethos in which medicine was practiced until recently, colleagues did not—apart from major ethical breaches—direct one another's behavior, nor were standards or protocols used to provide objective guidelines for care. Early managed care measures such as peer review, first used in the Medicare program, had minimal teeth and negligible influence on practice. The first versions of treatment plan preauthorization requirements and gatekeeper programs commonly gave rubber-stamp approvals for care.

Over time, managed care interventions grew bolder. Concomitant with assumption of control over reimbursement rates, payers' gained unprecedented influence over clinical decision making. For example, case managers today refuse to reimburse for unauthorized services, deny hospitalization requests, and influence hospital discharge dates (i.e., by denying reimbursement beyond a given day). Most payers have designed their own protocols to guide their managed care decisions. Although providers understandably are concerned that these protocols are biased toward cost efficiency rather than optimum care, few controlled clinical trials exist on which to base their designs. A new ethos for the practice of medicine has gradually emerged in which clinical decisions are no longer made exclusively at the bedside; physicians' decisions are reviewed by payer-employed peers.

The extent of cost savings from managed care is unclear, given the offset of substantial administrative costs. The new clinical and administrative roles for physicians and the relationship between clinicians and peer reviewers have more fundamental implications for medical practice than any cost reductions. Subsequent chapters consider the impact of the administrative physician on the role and behavior of the bedside physician, the potential ethical ramifications, the effects on the doctor-patient relationship, and other issues.

Most of the cost control measures just described have been applied to the mental health sector. Insurers have traditionally designed insurance benefits for mental health coverage more strictly than for general medical coverage, with "inside limits" including caps on the number of psychotherapy sessions and higher cost sharing requirements. Managed care is nearly universal among payers in their attempts to control mental health care costs. Many insurance companies manage mental health benefits separately under "carveout" arrangements that use more stringent financial and administrative measures to limit both supply of and demand for psychiatric services. As a result, the historical lack of parity for psychiatric care has persisted in the era of cost control, further widening the gap between mental health and general medical benefits.

Effects of Cost Control

United States health care expenditures continue to increase faster than the general inflation rate and to consume an ever higher percentage of gross domestic product (GDP). In 1994 (the most recent figures available), national health care spending was $938 billion and 13.9% of the national GDP (Burner and Waldo 1995). At the same time, the pace of health care expenditure increases has slowed significantly. Burner and Waldo project that health care costs will increase 8% annually between 1996 and 2005, compared to an average of 13.4% annually between 1973 and 1983. These numbers reflect the cumulative effect of the various public and private measures on supply and demand for medical care. It would be difficult to determine which cost control measures influenced this slowdown in growth most significantly, but PPS and managed care likely played essential roles.

Yet health care costs continue to elude predictability. Some analysts argue that because the product is health care, the supply- and demand-side measures described cannot fundamentally influence its use. Another major reason for the ongoing expenditure spiral is that reform measures to date have affected only one part of the health care system at a time. For every problem ameliorated (e.g., inpatient hospital costs), another problem has emerged (e.g., ambulatory and home health care costs), as partial reforms perpetuate the United States's nonsystem of health care.

If one accepts the assumption (which not all analysts will) that health care costs can be controlled, one theoretical model to achieve this end is comprehensive reform, such as creation of a universal, capitated insurance plan in a closed health care system with a global budget. Such a system spreads risk and eliminates the possibility of cost shifting, adverse selection, and public/private sector divisions. Its success would require supply-side financial and administrative incentives for efficient resource use, with personal and institutional accountability for quality and spending. HMOs and other organized systems of care begin to resemble in microcosm such a comprehensive system of care. They provide the opportunity to collect meaningful data for the analysis of long-term cost and health consequences of resource-use decisions, which would enable practitioners to learn how to optimize use of limited clinical resources.

But although such a plan is theoretically sound, it has proved impossible—for political and social reasons—to implement in the United States. Since the 1930s, Roosevelt and most subsequent presidents have considered national health policy reform, yet no proposal for comprehensive reform has passed into law. The most recent wave of national debate over major health policy reform occurred during the presidential campaign of 1992, and Clinton's election was due in part to his support for comprehensive reform. This failure to achieve congressional passage of such a plan reflected opposition from the insurance industry and organized medicine. As well, opinion polls indicated fear that such a plan would reduce patients' choice, disrupt physician relationships, and be poorly managed by the federal government.

The 1980s and Beyond— Emergence of a Volatile "Medical Marketplace"

The U.S. health care system is undergoing a dramatic transformation. Catalyzed and influenced initially by cost containment measures, by the mid-1990s the process had acquired independent momentum. Competition has been a major force for change, affecting all health care providers from hospitals to solo practitioners. This chapter concludes with a brief overview of: changes in the health care delivery system; effects on patients, physicians, and medical care; and issues arising from this new medical marketplace.

Several factors have catalyzed a downsizing of the hospital sector. Under managed care, hospitalization of every patient comes under scrutiny. Practitioners must justify and receive preapproval for their decisions to hospitalize patients, resulting in more conservative decisions to admit. In addition, new insurance benefit designs (e.g., PPS, capitation, rate negotiations) created incentives to move care out of the costly inpatient setting. Reflecting these changes, the average hospital occupancy rate, which had been steady at approximately 76% from 1960 through 1980, showed a marked decline in 1984, and in the late 1980s, it hovered at 66%. Because hospitalization generally is authorized only for acute, crisis-oriented treatment, the average length of stay has decreased markedly. Although the rate of hospital cost increases has slowed, the per-day costs have increased sharply, reflecting a resource-intensive stay for a more severely ill patient population.

As inpatient facility demand dwindled, many hospitals closed, merged, or were purchased by larger corporate entities. In 1989, there were 7% fewer hospitals than in 1979 and 5% fewer beds. From 1985 to 1987 alone, the number of hospital beds decreased almost 4% as a result of hospital closures and downsizings. In 1990, it was estimated that 12% of all hospitals were financially unstable and at ongoing risk.

In the public sector, efforts continue to shift the severely and persistently ill patient population out of asylums into community residential and treatment programs. The number of patients in asylums decreased from a peak population of 558,900 in 1955; today, long-stay residents in state mental hospitals number well under 100,000, with total bed capacity of about 107,000 (Manderscheid and Sonnenschein 1992). Despite the drop in resident population, state and county mental hospitals face a number of problems. Fiscal restraint leaves budgets inadequate for high-quality clinical programs. They must cope with high readmission rates because publicly supported aftercare services are lacking, resulting in the so-called revolving door syndrome (Sharfstein et al. 1995).

As care has shifted from hospitals to less costly settings, patient volume in outpatient practice sites has increased tremendously. In the mental health sector, the burgeoning ambulatory care sector includes psychiatric day hospitals, halfway houses and other residential programs, and in-home services. Although these outpatient sites are less expensive than the hospital, the growth in aggregate ambulatory expenditures is another example of cost shifting in the health care sector, offsetting any savings from reduced inpatient costs.

Success in today's entrepreneurial climate requires marketing skill to garner an adequate number of managed care contracts and the attendant patient volume. This shift of emphasis is evident: While the overall number of employees in the health care industry continues to grow, the number of employees in marketing, advertising, and public relations grew 71% over 6 years in the mid-1980s, whereas aides, orderlies, and attendants decreased by 27% during the same period.

Whereas health care itself was a profitable enterprise from the mid-1960s to the early 1980s, since that time the business of *constraining* health care resource use has become today's profitable health care industry. Managed care has become a growth industry, with public shareholders owning financial stakes in managed care companies that have become some of the most lucrative Wall Street investments available today. Although physicians, ethicists, and some policymakers deplore the fact that shareholders gain to the extent that managed care companies hold down the use of health care services, others argue that reductions in "waste" of health care resources merit every penny of profit.

Boundaries have become blurred between insurers, payers, and providers in the new medical marketplace, as the various entities assume new roles and responsibilities in an effort to maintain market shares or capture additional business. Some hospitals have capitalized on the shift to ambulatory care, surviving financially by transforming themselves into "health systems" offering a full continuum of services with the hospital at its organizational core. Some health systems now assume financial risk for care, sharing with employers or traditional insurers the role of insurer for large populations. In a more recent trend, physicians are forming single- or multispecialty groups that contract with employers or insurers to provide care for populations; such arrangements generally include shared financial risk. Managed care methods are critical to fiscal constraint in these new, "organized" systems of care.

Patients' experiences have changed. Marketplace innovations such as same-day surgery, preauthorization of benefits, and insurer case management have become commonplace. As costs of care become less affordable for the average family, more Americans than ever (in some United States markets, more than 50% of the population) are enrolling in HMOs and other organized systems of care (International Medical News Group 1996). Not only do such plans generally insure enrollees against catastrophic losses, often they also include preventive services while requiring minimal cost sharing. In return, however, patients may experience disruption of long-standing relationships with physicians and face administrative disincentives to seek care. In today's medical marketplace, however, relationships and convenience have been sacrificed to ensure affordability. Yet with lifetime limits, exclusions based on preexisting conditions, ever tightening standards of medical necessity, and variations in benefit design, even patients with seemingly good coverage experience serious deficits in coverage. Although physicians deplore these disruptions and the potentially reduced quality of care, surveys to date indicate high enrollee satisfaction with the care they receive in organized systems of care. Patient (or employer) discontent would be a likely stimulus to reform of current managed care practices; until patients become unhappy with their quality of care, these entities are likely to proceed as they do today. On a larger scale, "society" is unlikely to push for comprehensive system reform as long as individuals are satisfied with the quality and affordability of their health care.[2]

Physicians have experienced myriad changes as well, although we are only recently acknowledging their extent. We have traditionally been a fiercely independent group, priding ourselves on our relative immunity to social and political trends. This characteristic may explain why physicians showed minimal response to cost control measures for about the first 10 to 15 years of the cost control era. Perhaps convinced that cost control was a transient effort, physicians were late to modify their behavior in response to it. Yet managed care and the other effects of the cost crisis appear to be here to stay. Physicians may be learning that ignoring the process of health reform until is has been implemented has had deleterious effects on medical practice. Over the last few years, we have become more aware of the im-

---

[2]Notwithstanding the 40+ million Americans uninsured in the current system.

pact of public policy on the profession. Many have become proactive in the debate on health reform.

Yet even those who remain distant from the policy arena feel the effects of the new medical marketplace on their practices. Predominant sites of care have shifted from inpatient to ambulatory settings. Roles have changed as a new group of administrative and executive physicians collaborate in managed care ventures and oversee their clinical colleagues. With limited resources, discounted reimbursements, and threats of empty waiting rooms, many providers are negotiating prospective service contracts and shared financial risk with payers and insurers. They are learning to make do with fewer resources. Successful practice today requires of many physicians not only clinical skill and the ability to demonstrate efficiency and high-quality outcomes but also managerial skills and the ability to negotiate tenable contracts with payers and insurers.

To the extent that the administrative complexity and associated overhead required to meet the demands of managed care and regulatory agencies have increased, solo practice has become unwieldy. Many clinicians need the efficiencies and economies of scale to survive financially. Medical professionals are moving from solo practices to group practices or becoming employees of managed plans and networks. Medical practices are being purchased by hospitals that realize the importance of "owning" the clinicians.

Manpower trends reflect these changes. In 1978 there were an estimated 28,300 practicing psychiatrists in the United States. At that time, private office practice was the primary work setting of more than half of all psychiatrists, as well as a secondary work setting for 20% of them (Koran 1981). Results of a late 1980s survey of psychiatrists' professional settings suggested that younger psychiatrists "may have less opportunity to enter full-time private practice than they did in years past" (Olfson et al. 1994). Anecdotal evidence certainly supports this observation. Although the number of psychiatry residents has been stable in recent years, many psychiatrists are concerned by estimates projecting substantially reduced need for psychiatrists under managed health care. With the heightened stress in working conditions, declining reimbursements, fewer apparent opportunities for solo practice (a model traditionally coveted by psychiatrists), discouraged role models, and ever growing debt of medical school graduates, conditions may be ripening for a recruitment crisis in psychiatry.

Competition in the mental health sector is high, particularly regarding provision of psychotherapy. Nonphysician mental health care professionals who perform psychotherapy seek independent practitioner status through state licensing laws. Many heated political battles have occurred over legislative rights to provide these services; reflecting numerous legislative successes, psychotherapy now is reimbursable when performed by diverse professional types, including nurse practitioners, mental health counselors, social workers, marital and family therapists, and psychologists. The competitive arena has expanded to include privileges to prescribe medications, diagnose and/or treat independently, and hospitalize patients.

Modes of care have changed in other aspects of psychiatric care. Extended evaluation and observation of patients have become obsolete modes of practice. Another "luxury" is long-term psychotherapy, including psychoanalysis. Practitioners favoring these treatment approaches find themselves shut out of managed care panels that carefully profile physician practice styles.

Psychiatrists are treating most patients in ambulatory settings, using the continuum of care to treat patients with a wide range of clinical severities. In the process, psychiatrists are assuming greater legal risk as they treat even suicidal, psychotic, and low-functioning patients without the support of institutional settings and treatment teams. Facility with brief therapy models has become a necessary skill, as has provision of psychopharmacologic treatments in conjunction with nonphysician psychotherapists. Psychiatrists are learning to fare with fewer office visits and beginning to consider care in episodes of illness rather than long-term models, even for chronic illnesses. The overall tenor of practice has become more stressful as paperwork has increased, and telephone calls or written treatment plans have become mandatory before care is authorized. Physicians cope with gag rules and disrupted relationships—tradeoffs to maintain financial viability in the current market.

These changes reflect both the perils and the promise of the new marketplace. Along with the potential for improved clinical care as well as the opportunity to use data and practice protocols to improve quality of care comes the risk that valuable treatments will be discarded. Worse yet, the next generation of psychiatrists may not be trained in these time-tested models, risking their permanent loss.

Clearly, ethical issues are raised in this new medical marketplace. Autonomy, confidentiality, bedside clinical decision making—who is in charge? Whereas 20 or even 10 years ago, the answers were clear, today they are not. Lacking political and societal support and facing unprecedented financial hurdles, today's clinician lacks an unequivocal mandate to maintain his or her independence in clinical decision making. Yet as much as clinicians lament this loss of control, most are adapting to the frustration of today's administrative hurdles. More important than their personal discomfort over shrinking autonomy, however, is the concern of many practitioners that ever stricter cost control measures threaten their ability to provide patients with quality care. The challenge is to learn how to balance costs and care successfully.

The vocabulary has changed as hospitals have become "health systems," patients have become "consumers" or "clients," and doctors have become "providers"—has the "product" changed as well? Is medical care fundamentally different from the way it was 20 years ago? There is no simple answer to this seemingly straightforward question. Medical care is now provided in a competitive, cost-conscious, and heavily regulated environment. Yet we hope it has not fundamentally changed insofar as it is remains a one-on-one encounter between a person with a complaint regarding body or mind and a medical professional committed to help with that problem.

Where are we in 1998? Clearly, we are in a period of great instability as the financial and administrative underpinnings of practice continue to shift rapidly. Cost problems remain; despite all of the measures implemented during the last two decades, health care costs are still rising faster than general inflation. We are providing psychiatric care in a complex health care system facing ongoing pressures to reduce costs and struggling to maintain traditional values in an atmosphere of crisis. These issues resulting from our current circumstances will be explored in depth in subsequent chapters.

References

American Hospital Association: AHA Guide to the Health Care Field. Chicago, IL, American Hospital Association, 1990

Burner ST, Waldo DR: National health expenditure projections, 1994–2005. Health Care Financ Rev 16:221–242, 1995

Ellenberger HF: Psychiatry from ancient to modern times, in American Handbook of Psychiatry, 2nd Edition, Vol 1: The Foundations of Psychiatry. Edited by Arieti G. New York, Basic Books, 1974, pp 3–27

Foley HA, Sharfstein SS: Madness and Government: Who Cares for the Mentally Ill? American Psychiatric Press, Washington, DC, 1983

Frank RG, Salkever DS, Sharfstein SS: A new look at rising mental health insurance costs. Health Aff 10:116–123, 1991

International Medical News Group: Clinical Psychiatry News 24:1, 1996

Koran LM: Psychiatrists' distribution across the 50 states, 1978. Arch Gen Psychiatry 38:1155–1159, 1981

Manderscheid RW, Sonnenschein MA (eds): Mental Health: United States (Center for Mental Health Services DHHS Publ No SMA-92-1942). Washington, DC, U.S. Government Printing Office, 1992

National Center for Health Statistics: Health, United States, 1990. Hyattsville, MD, Public Health Service, 1991

Olfson M, Pincus HA, Dial TH: Professional practice patterns of U.S. psychiatrists. Am J Psychiatry 151:89–95, 1994

Sharfstein SS, Stoline AM, Koran LM: Mental health services, in Jonas's Health Care Delivery in the United States, 5th Edition. Edited by Kovner AR. New York, Springer, 1995, pp 232–266

Starr P: The Social Transformation of American Medicine. New York, Basic Books, 1982

Stoline AM, Weiner JP, Geller G, Gorovitz EK: The New Medical Marketplace: A Physician's Guide to the Health Care System in the 1990s, 2nd Edition. Baltimore, MD, Johns Hopkins University Press, 1993

White WA: Forty Years of Psychiatry. New York, Nervous and Mental Disease Publishing, 1933

CHAPTER TWO

Quality in Managed Care Systems: What Is in the Patient's Best Interests?

Alex R. Rodriguez, M.D.

In any pluralistic society, the competing interests of its citizens constantly test the architecture and constructs of its social values and legal systems. The very foundation of democratic institutions in the United States is based on late-eighteenth-century notions of the "divine right" of freedom of the individual citizen, with whom government has a social contract to uphold freedom from oppression and the relative freedoms of life, liberty, and the pursuit of happiness. These values have evolved with many fits and starts in such areas as civil rights. The evaluation of citizens' rights to health care, not explicitly ordained in the Constitution or Bill of Rights, has occurred through public initiatives such as the development of state hospital systems and entitlement programs (Medicare, CHAMPUS, Medicaid) and private initiatives such as health benefits and insurance. These initiatives have spawned government bureaucracies, private corporations, and other institutions with interests that have not only gone beyond the original purpose of helping meet the basic needs of citizens for quality health services, but in too many instances have also instituted competing agendas that interfere with the "best interests of the patient." In this chapter we will explore some of the issues that surround the needs of each citizen for health services that are accessible, affordable, low risk, and competent and that result in the highest possible health status.

Note: The views herein represent the personal opinions of the author and should not be construed to represent the views of Consortium Health Plans, Inc., the Department of the Navy, or the Department of Defense.

Current Contexts of Quality in Health Services

Defining and establishing quality in health care services is a dynamic process that changes over time, as the many forces that influence what quality is themselves undergo transformation. As the social values of American society have been shaped by enlightened views about sharing of common resources to meet common needs, so they have been dependent upon a strong economy that supports people's social and political goals. In attempting to fulfill the best interests of its citizens, the United States, the European community, and Japan represent a successful management of values with a viable economic system, whereas the former Soviet Union symbolizes a failure. The very strength of the American market economic system is its sensitivity to market forces. Both supply and demand are dependent upon a sound economy and the essential affordability of goods and services. The American economy is thus a major definer of what is both "right" and acceptable, relative to the needs of its people. The escalating absolute and relative costs of health services in the United States during the past 25 years have precipitated the current crisis in health care financing, which continues to seek viable means of cost restraints. This market environment has created managed care and now is organizing under health care reform measures to affect the way that all citizens receive health services.

The U.S. market economy, supported by an internationally competitive industrial and commercial might, has advanced the unforeseen expansion of health benefits to workers since the late 1940s through both private insurance and public entitlement programs. Budgets, bolstered by a combination of sales, taxes, and deficit borrowing, have sustained this growth, not appreciating that, in every society, there are periodic days of reckoning. For health care, that day has arrived. Employers and governments have concluded that health services are too freely available, costly, profitable, and unaccountable. Like its older android, utilization review, managed care has been created to deal with the "accountability problem" (Smith 1987). Their disquieting mood about costs of care notwithstanding, payers have been relatively restrained by counterbalancing market forces in their ambitions to rein in these costs:

Consumer Demand. Many employers continue to depend upon highly skilled employees to compete successfully in domestic and international markets. Because employees so highly value generous health benefits and access to high-quality health services, employers have learned to be sensitive to their demands. The role of unions and benefits consultants in educating employers about the gains in productivity that accrue with effective health services has been an important contributor to most benefits, including mental health, remaining intact as employers seek solutions to rising health care costs. Evolving consumerism is reflected in public polls and plan surveys that consistently indicate the importance of high-quality health services to citizens, the willingness of employees to shop for benefit plans that meet their needs for quality services, and the growing power of consumer advocacy groups that draw strength from conflicts over health benefits. The roles of consumers in influencing future policies of the legislative branches of governments, regulatory agencies, accreditation organizations (e.g., National Committee on Quality Assurance), and professional associations (e.g., American Psychiatric Association) will surely evolve further in defining and monitoring quality of care for consumers.

Legal Regulation. Few countries are more intrigued by the power of their legal system than the United States. This may explain in part why so many are attracted to practicing law, the public's fascination with the trial system, and the predisposition of citizens to utilize the tort system to redress grievances. Thus, health care is heavily influenced by legal actions and the threat of such actions. Utilization review, managed care, and states' efforts at health care reform have all been shaped by court decisions and other legal challenges. In the American way of doing things, this trend will surely continue, as courts further define the social contracts that exist between citizens and government, as well as other social institutions that have power over their freedoms. Although the inalienable right to quality health services was not explicitly promised by the framers of the Constitution and Bill of Rights, there seems to be little doubt that Americans consider a high level of health to be part of their entitlement to life, if not liberty and pursuit of happiness. This perceived collective now represents a formidable social value that will certainly be ethically affirmed and legally defined in future court decisions.

Scientific and Professional Determinations. Two of the consistently influential shapers of legal definitions of quality in health services are the scientific evidence of effectiveness of health care interventions and professional consensus about what constitutes appropriate care. As technical innovations have made health care in the United States the most advanced in the world, they have prolonged longevity and improved life functioning and satisfaction, while being supported by monumental infusions of cash from public and private sources, including health benefits funds. Americans have come to believe that their right to the "best" health care should provide them ready access to technologically sophisticated evaluations and treatments. In recent years, cost-effectiveness analysis and other epidemiological scientific approaches have increasingly been utilized to measure the efficacy of outcomes for individuals and populations. Technology and therapeutic assessment programs (e.g., Agency for Health Care Policy and Research, DATTA program of the American Medical Association) and practice parameters activities of national medical specialty organizations have sorted through the mass of scientific efficacy data to establish consensus about appropriate, "quality" health care. The weight of science in defining health benefits quality and equity is becoming very important in legal and ethical determinations about what is in the best interests of patients.

A number of additional contextual considerations are relevant to social consensus about patients' interests. First, there is common agreement that a major transformation is now under way in the United States with increasing valuation of communalistic social structures and a diminishing acceptance of individualistic values. Global economic and political changes have reduced the previous dominance and power of the U.S. economy to the point that economists are now seriously questioning the capacity of the American economic system to support the massive, governmentally supported infrastructure that has evolved over the past 60 years. The social value of supporting the greatest needs of the greatest numbers of citizens, within limited financial resources, is being embraced by American courts, government, and institutions. They are affirming that the "best" that society has to offer cannot be achieved by all, while struggling to define an acceptable standard of security that is affordable. The specter of rationing now looms over health care in debates over health care reform at the national and state levels. It is becoming more unclear each day to what extent the social contract between government and each citizen promises optimal health and social services. The gold standard of quality care would be met if positive health outcomes could be consistently achieved for defined health conditions (i.e., the highest possible patient functionality with the highest possible treatment satisfaction and life satisfaction). However, that ideal standard is not very often achieved because of limitations in geographical access, financial coverage, patient compliance, response to treatment, and other factors. The limitations in quality and availability of health services resulting from relatively diminishing financial resources has profound implications for public health, social stability and productivity, and scientific research and training (Rodriguez 1988).

The ethical context of responsibility to each patient is now creating a professional conundrum in defining roles of professional conduct within a changing and threatening economic milieu. Physicians are obligated by professional codes of ethics not to reject or otherwise discriminate against patients based solely on financial considerations, as well as to inform, assist, and not harm patients (American Psychiatric Association 1993; Clements 1992; Council on Ethical and Judicial Affairs 1994a, 1994b; Pellegrino 1981). Engelhardt and Rie (1989) have advocated that physicians should "tell the truth, . . . help people buy what they want, . . . make a profit, . . . love thy neighbor and be charitable, . . . honor, respect and advance the learned profession of medicine, and . . . market virtue, combining the provision of health services with a commitment to the rights and bests interests of patient." Sabin (1994) has established four principles he believes constitute a moral code for clinicians: 1) "As a clinician, I am dedicated to caring for my patients in a relationship of fidelity, and at the same time to acting as a steward of society's resources; 2) As a clinician, I believe it is ethically mandatory to recommend the least costly treatment unless I have substantial evidence that a more costly intervention is likely to yield a superior outcome; 3) In my stewardship role, I need to advocate for justice in the health care system, just as in my clinical role I need to advocate for the welfare of my patient; 4) If a potentially beneficial intervention does not meet the explicit public standards for third-party coverage in a just system, as a clinician I believe the ethical course is to withhold the intervention and to discuss the situation openly with my patient." He advocates that physicians not make idiosyncratic bedside decisions that may lead to patient-by-patient rationing and that they should instead participate in just, explicit, and public processes of rationing that constitute the future of "difficult choices" confronting practitioners, patients and their families, payers, and policymakers. Ultimately, it should be society's policy and each clinician's practice to actively promote the prevention of illness, the rapid and comprehensive treatment of acute medical episodes, and long-term treatment that supports the highest level of functioning and comfort for those with chronic conditions. In the moral and ethical contexts of practice, each clinician will need to address simultaneously the requests of the patient and family, the needs of the employer and community, one's own therapeutic capacities, and the rules of society in making treatment decisions. It is evident that many clinicians are struggling with this near-impossible balancing act.

A final context that shapes social consensus about patient needs and rights is the set of rules established by an individual patient's benefit plan. The tremendous variations in coverage, copayments, and rules governing access to care are major contributors to variations in health status and quality of the health care process and outcomes across the United States and a significant point in the argument for health care reform. Common "rules" should govern universality of access, benefit coverage, payment, and other issues relevant to parity and justice in health services. This would fulfill society's communalistic strivings. However, individuals with their own strivings for the best care, rather than that which is commonly good, represent a force that will constantly interject the wholly American notion of individual freedom into the public debate about rightness in health services. Thus, the insurance or entitlement contract established by the health plan will most certainly continue to vary from individual to individual, depending upon their economic worth as much as their political rights. In this sometimes troubling and confusing period where society is struggling with the moral dilemmas caused by individual freedom, economic limits, and inequality, health care reform is also struggling to birth. The failure of the 103rd Congress to enact health care reform legislation dramatized the complexity of setting rules about benefit coverage that can be fair to all, affordable, clearly definable, and consistently provided. The ethical concerns reflected in the health care reform mission will definitively add to the complexities of program design, implementation, administration, financing, and monitoring (Council on Ethical and Judicial Affairs 1994a). They also are poised to contribute to one of the potentially great successes in U.S. history.

Defining Quality

Quality, as much as any explainable condition, has as many definitional constructs as there are people who have an opinion about it. A popular explanation paraphrases U.S. Supreme Court Justice Potter Stewart's notion of pornography: "I may not know how to define it, but I know it when I see it." For this chapter on quality issues, a current and widely quoted definition by the Institute of Medicine at the National Academy of Sciences (1993) is cited. "Quality of care . . . is the degree to which health services for individuals and populations increase the likelihood of desired health outcomes and are consistent with current knowledge." Health benefits policies commonly define quality in terms of "medical necessity," that is, health services that

- are adequate and essential for the evaluation or treatment of a medical disease, illness, or condition as defined by standard diagnostic nomenclatures (ICD-9CM [Medicode Inc. 1994] or DSM-IV [American Psychiatric Association 1994]);
- can reasonably be expected to improve an individual's condition or level of functioning;
- are in keeping with national standards of health professional practice as defined by standard clinical references and valid empirical experience for efficacy of services; and
- are provided in the most cost-effective manner and at the most cost effective level of care.

Health services researchers define quality in terms of measurable components of health status improvement, cost-effectiveness, and adverse occurrences. The movement toward outcomes measurement is rapidly evolving as a megatrend in health care to the point that almost all health care payers and providers are either implementing outcomes monitoring programs or considering an implementation strategy. A significant component of current outcomes monitoring involves the assessment of patient satisfaction with health care medical and administrative services and the correlation of this satisfaction with functional status and general life satisfaction. The popularization of continuous quality improvement (CQI) programs in health care reinforces this patient-centric focus on quality assessment, deriving from its ethic of treating patients as a valued source of information in order to improve service to them. In surveying patients, a number of attributes of quality health care consistently surface, relative to what they consider to be in their best interests. These could be referred to as the "10 Cs" of quality for patients.

- *Competence:* technical skills of all health care professionals providing care
- *Caring:* compassion, empathy
- *Convenience:* rapid access to skilled care, with administrative ease
- *Comfort:* physical surroundings conducive to healing and relief of pain and discomfort
- *Continuity:* consistency of competent care over time
- *Conscientiousness:* adhering to ethical practices
- *Communications:* effective explanations and education, with clearly defined informed consent
- *Coordination:* effective connection of components of evaluation and treatment with administration of services
- *Cooperativeness:* clear commitment to work with the patient to achieve health
- *Cost-effectiveness:* Sensitivity to costs of care to the patient, correlated to effective outcomes

In attempting to provide quality of care to patients and their families, providers and managed care organizations (MCOs) should also be cognizant of the importance of these same 10 factors to employers. As payers of health care services and because of concerns about work productivity and the welfare of the employee, employers want accountability for their investments in health benefits. A positive change in employers' attitudes and approaches to this accountability is their increasing interest in considering employees, providers, and MCOs as their partners. The view that all parties share the responsibility for cost-conscious, quality health services is an outgrowth of the CQI movement and the trend toward communalistic responses to shared problems. The increased mutual dialogue has resulted in joint planning, programming, and performance monitoring that seek to develop more creative means of supporting the occupational-business mission of the employer and the needs of employees. This increasing move toward collaboration is an important trend in the market reform of health care services.

Structuring Quality in Health Services

Achieving quality in the process and outcome of care is the primary shared goal of each patient and provider. In meeting the ethical requirements for promoting the positive health outcome of the patient (beneficence) while not causing harm (nonmaleficence), the provider assumes responsibility for establishing and managing systems that will best ensure that quality care is provided (McCullough 1993). The structures for quality management in direct patient care have evolved during the twentieth century in the United States through many initiatives directed at quality in the institutional setting and in the training, supervision, licensure, certification, and performance monitoring of individual practitioners. The structures of health care delivery systems promote quality through the provision of clinical staff that are competent, available in adequate numbers and disciplines, and supported by adequate diagnostic and therapeutic resources and administrative supports such as clinical policies and patient care databases. Provider legal exposure is established by risks to patients of adverse outcomes when these quality structures, processes, and outcomes are not in place or functioning. Accreditation programs established by independent national organizations (e.g., National Committee for Quality Assurance, Joint Commission on Accreditation of Healthcare Organizations), state and federal agencies (e.g., CHAMPUS), and private MCOs attempt to validate the effective functioning of these structures. Although the preponderance of these efforts is seemingly defensive (i.e., trying to prevent injury and legal exposure), a substantial amount of effort is directed at the professional mission of caring. Organizations that effectively convey commitment to the patient as a person often also prosper, so quality caring can also serve the offensive objective of success in the health services market. CQI approaches that promote the positive quest for quality now seem well on their way to becoming an elemental part of direct care delivery systems (Batalden 1993).

These quality management systems at the direct care level provide a major foundation for patient care quality needs in managed care systems. Among the major reasons that payers and patients have found managed care attractive are managed care's quality management structures that enhance coordination, cost-effectiveness, and, in some instances, the competence of care. Responsible managed care organizations are quality driven, service oriented, and sensitive to ethical issues. MCOs are struggling with conflict-of-interest concerns related to the split fiduciary roles they serve for the patient, themselves, and the MCO (Hillman 1987; Pellegrino 1986; Petrila and Cotler 1994; Povar and Moreno 1988; Relman 1988). They have also struggled to be sensitive to the unique needs for confidentiality, continuity, and access that persons with mental disorders present (Becker, et al. 1992; Blum 1992; Sabin and Sharfstein 1994; Schreter 1993; Wilson 1985). Although some specialty managed behavioral health organizations (MBHOs) have generally provided a higher level of access to medically necessary mental health and substance abuse care than full-service MCOs (HMOs, PPOs), providers and patients continue to experience difficulties with MBHOs' oversight roles and procedures, service functions (e.g., phone availability, claims payment), reimbursements, and clinical protocols. There are many current concerns about the impact of managed care on graduate mental health professional training due to reimbursement policies that limit payment to trainees (Blackwell and Schmidt 1992).

Notwithstanding these problems striving for solutions, MBHOs have generally satisfied employers, unions, and patients that they are committed to helping patients and their families receive quality mental health care. Payers clearly believe this enhanced accountability of quality, costs, and risks is worth the additional administrative fees of MBHOs and the reduced absolute freedom of choice available in indemnity programs. They and knowledgeable benefits consultants are constantly refining the service specifications for MBHO quality management and reporting functions, emphasizing the need for science-based clinical protocols, case management by skilled mental health professionals, and comprehensive integrated mental health networks. The hunger by employers and MCOs for data on quality and cost outcomes of these investments is driving them toward further investments in data systems that will provide more sophisticated conclusions about the cost-effectiveness and appropriateness of health care services. An example of such a collaborative effort between employers, consumers, and MCOs is the Health Plan Employer Data and Information Set (HEDIS 3.0), developed by the National Committee for Quality Assurance (1997). The development of practice profile systems is envisioned as an opportunity to improve on provider, patient, and delivery systems variables that impact upon quality health outcomes. Closely allied to such clinical management systems will be targeted CQI activities, professional and patient education programs, structured technology and therapeutic assessment functions, and refinements in practice parameters. Employers are also seeing MCOs as their partners in offering worksite health promotion and disease prevention services, employee assistance services, and integrated occupational-environmental health management. Their need for integrated benefits management will ultimately link now diversely managed employee benefits, disability, and workers' compensations benefit activities under full-service MCOs. This integration, envisioned and planned under various health care reform proposals, will serve the common needs of employers and employees to promote optimal productivity, job satisfaction, and life satisfaction through the prevention of illness and promotion of health.

What continues to remain unclear is the role of government in promoting quality health outcomes. The political counterposition of a federal government that boldly envisions a major reorganization in health services nationally while declaring that Diagnosis-Related Groups, and not managed care, are the solution for the ills of Medicare seems very contradictory. Although there are many questions about commitments (Chassin 1993) and solutions (Berwick 1994) to quality management under federal health care reform, the Clinton Administration should at least be lauded for the leadership that focused the nation and its legislative representatives on a long-standing crisis that will require national changes and sacrifices if the United States is ever to establish justice in health care services. The need for national leadership in developing systems of outcomes management (Ellwood 1988) remains very high, but the ability and reduced popular mandate of the federal government to drive the level of change needed to ensure quality health services for all citizens seem fairly limited. Change is occurring dramatically for Medicaid-borne universal access in a number of states such as Oregon, Tennessee, and Hawaii, but the problems in setting up such programs is great (Hadorn 1991). The irresistible force of adding large numbers of persons with expensive health care needs does not seem to budge the immovable object of tax-limited budgets without great friction. Ultimately, level-headed people begin to soberly rationalize the rightness of rationing care, while hoping "quality" can be preserved (Eddy 1994). Yet the question remains: How can governments spend so much of their resources on so many questionable allocations and not consider the health and welfare of its citizens to be worth more than what rationing will allow? Although rationing currently occurs unfairly because of financial and other impediments to access, is it any fairer to deny bone marrow transplantation or meaningful mental health services to a person because cost-effectiveness analysis, policy boards, and other socially sanctioned due process systems deem such individuals to be of lesser worth to society? These are vexing questions that underscore the truly critical answers that will define just how great or limited the morality of U.S. civilization will be in the twenty-first century. In the ethos of modern civilization, the social contract between citizen and government should be based on the same principles that define any healthy relationship: 1) trust, based on shared commitments to standards of fair play and the "golden rule," 2) mutual respect, 3) open and complete expressions of thinking and feeling, 4) timely follow-through on written and verbal obligations, and 5) a shared interest and obligation to help one another. That citizens seem less committed to supporting their governments and other traditional institutions may be less attributable to a culture of narcissism than the problems those institutions have had in promoting loyalty through listening to the needs of the people they were created to serve. In the next epoch of change in health care, the institutions that fulfill the deep moral need of people for commitment to their welfare will frame a new social contract dedicated to the individual and collective right of all citizens for quality health and social services. The legacy of this future is being determined by the ethics of the present.

References

American Psychiatric Association: The Principles of Medical Ethics—With Annotations Especially Applicable to Psychiatry. Washington, DC, American Psychiatric Association, 1993

American Psychiatric Association: Diagnostic and Statistical Manual of Mental Disorders. Washington, DC, American Psychiatric Association, 1994

Batalden P: The continual improvement of health care. Am J Med Qual 8:29–31, 1993

Becker J, Tiano L, Marshall S: Legal issues in managed mental health, in Managed Mental Health Care. Edited by Fitzpatrick R, Feldman JL. Washington, DC, American Psychiatric Press, 1992, pp 159–183

Berwick DM: Eleven worthy aims for clinical leadership of health system reform. JAMA 272:797–802, 1994

Blackwell B, Schmidt GL: The educational implications of managed mental health care. Hosp Community Psychiatry 43:962–964, 1992

Blum SR: Ethical issues in managed mental health, in Managed Mental Health Services. Edited by Feldman S. Springfield, IL, Charles C Thomas, 1992, pp 245–265

Chassin M: The missing ingredient in health reform—quality of care. JAMA 270:377–378, 1993

Clements CD: Systems ethics and the history of medical ethics. Psychiatr Q 63:367–390, 1992

Council on Ethical and Judicial Affairs, American Medical Association: Ethical issues in health care system reform. JAMA 272:1056–1062, 1994a
Council on Ethical and Judicial Affairs, American Medical Association: Ethics guidelines for managed care (Report 13-A-94). Chicago, IL, American Medical Association, 1994b
Eddy DM: Rationing resources while improving quality. JAMA 272: 817–824, 1994
Ellwood PM: Outcomes management: a technology of patient experience. N Engl J Med 318:1549–1556, 1988
Engelhardt HT Jr, Rie MA: Morality for the medical-industrial complex. N Engl J Med 319:1086–1089, 1989
Hadorn DC: Setting health care priorities in Oregon: cost effectiveness meets the rule of the rescue. JAMA 265:2218–2225, 1991
Hillman AL: Financial incentives for physicians in HMOs: is there a conflict of interest? N Engl J Med 317:1743–1748, 1987
Institute of Medicine: Washington, DC, National Academy of Sciences, 1993
McCullough LB: Ethics in the management of health care organizations. Physician Exec 19:72–76, 1993
National Committee for Quality Assurance: HEDIS 3.0. Washington, DC, National Committee for Quality Assurance, 1997
Pellegrino ED: Rationing health care: the ethics of medical gatekeeping. J Contemp Health Law Policy 2:23–45, 1986
Pellegrino, ED, Thomasma DC: A Philosophical Basis of Medical Practice. New York, Oxford University Press, 1981, pp 207–219
Petrila J, Cotler M: Ethical hazards to capitation contracting: legal and ethical concerns. Behav Healthc Tomorrow 3:41, 45–46, 1994
Povar G, Moreno J: Hippocrates and the health maintenance organization: a discussion of ethical issues. Ann Intern Med 109:419–424, 1988
Relman AS: Salaried physicians and economic incentives. N Engl J Med 319:784, 1988
Rodriguez AR: An introduction to quality assurance in mental health, in Handbook of Quality Assurance in Mental Health. Edited by Stricker G, Rodriguez AR. New York, Plenum, 1988, pp 26–27
Sabin JE: A credo for ethical managed care in mental health practice. Hosp Community Psychiatry 45:859–860, 1994
Sabin JE, Sharfstein SS: Ethical issues in managed care, in Allies and Adversaries: The Impact of Managed Care on Mental Health Services. Edited by Schreter RK, Sharfstein SS, Schreter CA. Washington, DC, American Psychiatric Press, 1994, pp 187–200

Schreter RK: Ten trends in managed care and their impact on the biopsychological model. Hosp Community Psychiatry 44:325–327, 1993

Smith MAH: Accountable in any system. American Medical News 30:4, 1987

Wilson GF: Ethical and legal aspects of peer review, in Psychiatric Peer Review: Prelude and Promise. Edited by Hamilton JM. Washington, DC, American Psychiatric Press, 1985, pp 57–70

Section II
Roles for Psychiatrists in the New Medical Marketplace

CHAPTER THREE

Psychiatrists and the New Managed Systems of Care: Roles and Responsibilities

Lloyd I. Sederer, M.D.

We are at a moment in the history of American medicine where the financing of care is the preeminent force shaping the service delivery system. Morreim put it most succinctly: "[E]conomics is rewriting medicine" (Morreim 1990)." At an astonishing velocity, the refinancing of health care—especially mental health care—principally through the phenomenon of "managed care," is refashioning a century of medical traditions and practices (Enthoven 1980; Sederer and Bennett 1996; Tischler 1990). For physicians, professional and personal lives are inextricably tied to the restructuring of health care, and its impact already is profoundly felt. For psychiatrists who trained more than 10 or 15 years ago and for those medical students drawn to psychiatry for its emphasis on the mind, reflection, and the doctor-patient relationship, the heart and soul of the field appears endangered. The solo office practice of dynamic psychiatry may become one of the first casualties of health reform.

Many of our colleagues are deeply pained and frightened by the direction our field has taken. How will the practice of psychiatry remain a source of professional and personal satisfaction? Evidence is growing that managed care per se, at least for nonpsychiatric physicians, does not preclude satisfaction (Baker and Cantor 1993; Reames and Dunstone 1989; Schultz et al. 1992). No published reports exist to date on the satisfaction of psychiatrists in managed mental health care. However, a recent survey of the membership of the Massachusetts Psychiatric Society indicates that satisfaction correlates highly with professionally challenging and stimulating work and the utilization of valuable skills (Sederer et al. 1994). How can psychiatry meet the economic mandate without compromising its intellectual foundations and the professional satisfaction essential to sustain its practitioners and recruit its future members? Can this be done in the face of intense and unrelenting economic forces?

This chapter first suggests why we should not be fully persuaded by notions of the medical marketplace or the corporatization of medicine. However, though the practice of psychiatry may not be a business, the provision of psychiatric services, especially to insured populations, will have to be conducted in a businesslike manner. The chapter then discusses two roles essential to psychiatric practice in managed systems of care. Unless psychiatrists function as experts and employers, the care patients require and the protection our field warrants may be vulnerable to erosion by architects of cost containment and service redesign. The chapter concludes with a perspective on past reformations in psychiatry and on the role of leadership.

The Medical Marketplace

The reform of health care in the United States became a political and economic necessity by the early 1990s. Despite a steep ascent in health care spending, far in excess of the nation's economic growth, the availability and affordability of medical insurance and services, especially for the middle class, was growing elusive. Cost-shifting was commonplace. Business and government were increasingly concerned about the "budget busting" threat of health care. Managed care and managed competition, through organized, competing systems of care in a reformed marketplace, have been put forward as a principal solution to the health care crisis (e.g., the Clinton Health Security Act of 1993). But to "largely entrust cost containment to the nebulous dynamics of prudent consumer shopping in a little reformed marketplace" seems a very large step for this country (Brown 1994).

Try as some may, with due respect to economics and competition, the "marketplace" analogy does not adequately encompass medical care (Annas 1993; Fein 1986; Stoline and Weiner 1988). Current attempts to industrialize medicine face many problems. It is one thing to wait in line for a movie. It is another thing to wait in line for a hip replacement or admission to a psychiatric hospital for acute suicidality. As Annas put it, evidently quoting the American Medical Association, Americans "would rather sue than queue" (Annas 1993, p. 213). Yet a practice environment of diminishing resources puts physicians in the role of allocating scarce resources, a role at variance with traditional medical ethics in which the individual patient comes first. Mechanic regarded this as a shift from "advocacy to allocation," which will further test the trustworthiness of the doctor-patient relationship (Mechanic 1986; Thompson 1992). Moreover, patients simply do not possess a full knowledge of alternatives—as do educated consumers of other services—and when in distress do not seek bargains. Finally, we are far from a market where financial savings would be returned to the consumers, which is one reason Enthoven maintained that managed care heretofore has failed to contain costs (Enthoven 1993). Though aspects of a "marketplace" exist, medicine differs from industry. Fein was probably correct in maintaining that health care policy is closer to social than to economic policy (Fein 1986, p. v).

Yet even when finances clearly drive an organization, physicians and other clinicians are host to more complex sources of motivation (Greco and Eisenberg 1993; Kahn 1993; Sederer 1994). Personal concerns, academic ambitions, practice environment, autonomy, achievement, satisfaction, social responsibility, and recognition are among the many motivators shaping physician behavior. Furthermore, physicians hold a deep conviction that their self-regard should rest on a foundation of quality care. Compromising care hence brings with it a diminishment in personal esteem and integrity. Physicians cannot—and should not—tolerate care they regard as less than optimal because of the professional and personal consequences.

Physicians also experience what Morreim has called "new duties in the medical standard of care" (Morreim 1991). Specifically, the physician, she argues, has an obligation to disclose to the patient their costs, any financial incentives under which the physician (or organized system of care) is operating, as well as the generally accepted standards of medical care. In effect, under these duties the physician is obligated to inform his or her patient of the manifold and competing interests inherent in medical decision making. This obligation is also likely to support a professional model of medicine and curtail its commodification.

Efforts to corporatize medicine will also be limited by the enormous regulatory environment that grips medical practice. Hospitals and clinics must be certified by a host of state and national, private and public organizations and agencies. Physicians must be licensed, credentialed, and continuously educated. Every payer and managed care organization has its membership standards and "quality" measures. For the most part, regulation was conceived and introduced to protect the public interest. The medical marketplace simply cannot extract itself from decades of regulatory control and operate as if it were in a relatively free marketplace.

Regulatory demands are reinforced by the needs, wishes, and expectations of patients, families, and advocacy groups. As ethical and elegant as population-based managed care may sound, virtually no physician has seen a patient or family compromise their own care for the community good or for a more "worthy" disorder. Professional practice will succeed only when it attends to those whom it services, namely patients and families (with the possible exception of government-run services for the destitute, disabled, or incarcerated).

The limits of the marketplace notwithstanding, medicine in general (and psychiatry as well) has no choice but to conduct itself in a businesslike manner. Nothing short of an explicit demonstration of value and accountability will result in the proper allocation of dollars and services for health care. If psychiatrists are to determine their future, there are two principal roles essential to doing so in the emerging managed system of care.[1] These are the roles of the psychiatrist as expert and employer.

---

[1] From the 1930s until the early 1970s, payment for psychiatric services was out of pocket and supported a significant ambulatory care system, especially for psychotherapeutic services. We may see a return of fee-for-service, out-of-pocket purchase of services as patients seek the privacy and intensity of care that seems unlikely in managed systems of care. Nevertheless, the primary site of insured psychiatric care, especially for major mental disorders, will likely be in organized systems of care. The discussion that follows addresses the roles and responsibilities of psychiatrists choosing to work, at least part-time, in those settings.

Psychiatrists as Experts

As experts, psychiatrists must seek to maintain legitimate authority. No other specialty group—mental health or medical—has been trained and exposed to the etiology, pathogenesis, course, treatments, and outcome of all mental disorders. The extent to which care will be effectively, efficiently, and economically provided will rely heavily on the expertise of psychiatrists. And the training and experience necessary to warrant expertise is more formidable as knowledge grows. Moreover, knowledge of the science of the brain and the body is not sufficient. A fundamental understanding of the mind, the personality, and human development remains critical in recognizing and treating illness and dysfunctional behavior. There are no shortcuts to obtaining that knowledge: Gifted teachers, long hours with patients, and a personal therapy or psychoanalysis remain the touchstones for anyone who seeks more than a superficial understanding of human nature and its sufferings.

Primary Tasks

The primary tasks for psychiatrists functioning as experts are likely to be defining and delivering quality care; fostering patient and family satisfaction; and providing training and supervision (Berwick 1989; Donabedian 1985; Fink 1993; Sederer 1991). Quality has been defined as that which "consistently contributes to the maintenance or improvement of health and well-being" (American Medical Association 1989). Quality has traditionally been assessed along three dimensions: structure, process, and outcome. More recently, quality has been considered in its technical and relational components (McGlynn et al. 1988). Technical aspects of quality refer to the procedures and treatments rendered and their outcomes; relational aspects of quality refer to the humane aspects of medical care including the doctor-patient relationship, respect, thoughtfulness, kindness, and caring. When surveyed, patients note these as separate dimensions of quality and weigh each significantly.

Satisfaction is related to quality but is not fully congruent. A patient may be unsatisfied with an effective treatment that was properly (technically) rendered. A patient may also be satisfied despite an unfortunate outcome (Eisen et al. 1991). Assessment and improvement of patient and family satisfaction are already becoming fundamental measures of health services and may find their way onto the "report cards" of the future.

Primary Tools

The primary tools of psychiatrists as experts will be their knowledge and experience; outcomes-oriented databases and practice parameters; and "consumer" (patient and family) surveys. Surveys will provide an opportunity to obtain the patient's perspective; as previously noted, technical and humane aspects of patient care are quality measures that also can be measured. Systems of psychiatric care are likely to be required to report on, and respond to, satisfaction information derived from ongoing assessment. In fact, retention in networks of care may have as one criterion the satisfaction ratings by the patient on clinicians who care for them.

In everyday practice, we are already at the outset of the utilization of symptom and functional assessment instruments and practice guidelines (Kassirer 1994; Relman 1988; Sederer 1991). Self-administered, optically scanned, and computer-analyzed reports of clinical outcomes and patient satisfaction are likely to become standard practice within several years and will serve as the basis for continuously updating practice guidelines and patient-oriented services (see also chapter 8). Psychiatrists as experts should take a leading role in this area if they are to influence their futures. Rapid access to information, continuous learning, and active participation in reshaping patient care practices will be characteristic of professional practice in a managed system of care.

Service Sites: Mental Health Sites

The provision of psychiatric services in the new managed system of care is likely to occur in two principal locations: in mental health and in primary care practice sites. In mental health service sites the specific skills and responsibilities of the psychiatrist, his or her relative scarcity and cost, and the liability inherent in the physician's role may insist that the psychiatrist provide or oversee the initial assessment, diagnosis, formulation, and treatment plan. This is far more than a gatekeeper role. Psychiatrists will have an opportunity to become expert leaders of a team of professionals. In a managed system of care, the psychiatrist would personally determine 1) the diagnosis (along all five axes); 2) the formulation (What vulnerabilities have been stressed by what current circumstances to prompt the dysfunction that spurs the patient to seek help?); 3) a plan for establishing an alliance with the patient and critical others; 4) a treatment plan that sequences needed care; and 5) recommendations as to who will be providing which aspects of care. Patients returning for care after a period of time will require the same vigorous, psychiatrist-led assessment and treatment planning.

For patients who then continue in care, the role of the psychiatrist in an organized system with multidisciplinary professional teams (at every level of care) becomes more limited and focused. Those services that only the psychiatrist can render, or is best prepared to provide, are likely to occupy his or her attention for both quality and cost considerations. Especially critical will be biomedical care, consultation, supervision, clinical administration, and leadership.

Biomedical care refers to biological and somatic assessments and treatments as well as liaison with other physicians. Obviously this includes the prescription of psychoactive medications, though we can anticipate that master's level clinical nurse specialists will provide some of this service in collaboration with a supervising psychiatrist. But psychopharmacology is only part of the psychiatrist's role. The psychiatrist will need to identify and conceptually integrate psychiatric, substance abuse, mental retardation, and medical comorbidities. The psychiatrist will have to "lay on hands," prepared to assess the patient physically if needed. Laboratory testing, imaging, radiologic, electroencephalographic, and electrocardiographic studies will be important (and expensive) assessments that the psychiatrist must order, evaluate, and act upon. Electroconvulsive therapy and light treatments are other biomedical aspects of psychiatric care that will be within the psychiatric domain.

For ongoing patients, even those not receiving biomedical interventions, psychiatric consultation will be essential for patients, families, and nonpsychiatric mental health practitioners. The art and science of consultation is likely to become a more necessary skill for the psychiatric resident to learn before entering managed systems of care. Diagnostic and treatment consultation for patients, families, and colleagues should be readily provided. It is better to respond to these requests than to question their utility. Consultations may focus upon the accuracy of the diagnosis and the formulation, on the alliance, the countertransference, environmental forces destabilizing the patient or the treatment (e.g., homelessness, illness, or loss of a loved one, financial problems limiting acquisition of medications), the appropriateness of the biological or psychosocial psychiatric treatments, or complicating medical problems. Consultations are optimal when they inform all those seeking help (the patient, the practitioner, the family, and, at times, the payer). Consultations support good treatment, improve care whenever possible, aid in risk management, and provide hope to all those engaged in a demanding or protracted treatment.

Finally, the clinical administration of mental health services, especially acute or intensive care, appears to be a vital and expanding role for the psychiatrist, again for both quality and cost considerations. Chapters by Drs. Axelson and Geraty elaborate on this point. In order to bring our expertise fully to bear on the care provided, psychiatrists ought not to shy away from clinical administration. Clinical administration merges clinical training, group and systems understanding, the scientific method, economic and business capabilities, and leadership skills. In the best of times, clinical administration can be a source of professional satisfaction for psychiatrists. In difficult times, psychiatric administration may provide considerably less satisfaction but becomes critically important in maximizing the care provided to patients and, consequently, professional and personal satisfaction.

Service Sites: Primary Care

The primary care practice of medicine has long represented a vast and underserved opportunity area. The success of fully integrated (i.e., medical/surgical/mental health/rehabilitative) systems of care, especially those capitated for all services, will rely on the prevention and early detection of psychiatric illness and on effective treatments woven into the everyday delivery of primary care. Primary care physicians estimate that a significant proportion of office visits are related to psychiatric or substance abuse problems. Emergency care and unnecessary and costly diagnostics often result when psychiatric diagnoses and treatment are not properly rendered.

Psychiatric services may be written into primary care practice guidelines. For example, a psychiatrist might "cotreat" a common primary care disorder (e.g., depression) by meeting conjointly with the patient and the primary care physician at frequent intervals in order to ensure proper diagnosis and adequate treatment (type, dose, and duration) throughout the course of the illness (Katon 1993). Short of cotreatment is the existing practice of constituting multispecialty group practices in which, for example, a family practitioner, pediatrician, obstetrician-gynecologist, psychiatrist (and often a psychologist or social worker), and perhaps one or two other physicians provide comprehensive services to a large panel of patients. In a multispecialty group practice the psychiatrist provides assessment and consultation as well as ongoing care for patients under the care of the other specialists or for those specifically referred to the psychiatric practice. Perhaps we can anticipate a future in which psychiatric and behavioral medicine services become an important aspect of population-based health management. After all, untreated psychiatric illnesses, habit disorders, and addictions are responsible for many of the ailments and functional impairments (and medical expenses) of middle and late life.

Challenges to Psychiatric Expertise

Psychiatrists serving as experts will face a panoply of difficulties and dilemmas. Practice guidelines may offer a basis for shaping effective treatments, supporting reimbursement, and aiding in risk management but are only in their infancy. Current guidelines tend to be consensus statements that preserve some of the complexity, variation, and art of practice. We can anticipate more specific algorithms or decision trees as practice-based outcome measurements improve but with a potential loss of breadth and creativity. For now, however, guidelines and outcomes-oriented care offer only limited tools in establishing the parameters for managed care and in supporting psychiatric expertise.

Psychiatrists as experts likely will bear the principal clinical responsibility for care in managed systems. However, authority over that care may be more elusive. When team practices characterize the provision of care, the psychiatrist will have to earn the role of team captain. Leadership is never achieved merely by designation or through organizational charts. Authority and leadership are truly obtained the old-fashioned way: They are earned. Those psychiatrists who know every facet of illness and remediation (as well as adaptation) are the ones likely to gain the credibility needed to attain actual authority. And psychiatrists who become experts in the economics, financing, and delivery of services will be better able to achieve leadership and success in practice groups and in the new managed systems of care.

Liability is of increasing concern to practicing psychiatrists. Practitioners are exposed to liability when a breach exists between those who provide care and those who pay (Appelbaum 1993; McCormick 1994). The psychiatrist's predicament may be that of recommending a specific treatment plan only to have that plan denied payment by a third or fourth party that controls the funds. Two dangers exist. The first danger is an adverse outcome if care is not provided, leaving the patient harmed and the psychiatrist at risk for a malpractice claim. The second danger, if the psychiatrist forcefully advocates for the patient, is to be "delisted" (i.e., dropped from the managed care network or denied future referrals). When medical and financial responsibility are integrated, rather than decoupled by "carve-out" companies, closer congruence between clinical and financial goals can exist because there will be no escape from ongoing responsibility for the patient.

Competition is yet another payer force that is likely to challenge psychiatrist expertise in managed systems of care. Now occurring between primary care physicians and psychiatrists, competition has a long history among the mental health disciplines. With limited budgets and financial disincentives to refer to specialists, primary care physicians are apt to be reluctant to hand off to psychiatrists those patients whom they believe they can treat. The recognition and treatment of psychiatric disorders in primary care, however, is less than optimal (Kessler et al. 1985; Narrow et al. 1933; Ormel et al. 1993; Wells et al. 1994). Underdiagnosis and undertreatment are common in primary care, and specialty referrals too often await late-stage disease progression. These factors limit the patient's clinical response and adversely affect the psychiatrist's ability to demonstrate effectiveness. Between psychiatrists and other mental health practitioners, the years have intensified competition and prompted some remarkable examples of cooperation. If psychiatrists become more medically identified and if psychologists and social workers desist from attempts to assume traditional medical responsibilities, greater cooperation may be possible. Cooperation notwithstanding, the absolute numbers of mental health practitioners, especially in many urban areas, represent an oversupply that is likely to sustain rather fierce competition in the foreseeable future.

Psychiatrists as Employers

Financial, medicolegal, and clinical risks appear to be the unavoidable requisites of psychiatric leadership in the new managed systems of care. To abrogate these responsibilities to other professional disciplines or to those exclusively trained in finance or management is to place our patients and profession in greatest jeopardy. If we are persuaded that we can best represent our patients and ourselves, the best way to do so is to successfully compete for that responsibility.

Currently, physician decisions result in approximately 75% of all medical service costs (Ginzberg 1992). Moreover, in 1993, one fifth of American acute-care hospitals had established corporate physician practice organizations. The remaining hospitals tended to be smaller, were not organized systems of care, and, in substantial numbers, were planning to develop a physician-hospital organization (Ernst & Young 1993). Physician-hospital organizations (PHOs) are becoming a primary means for aligning the financial interests of doctors and hospitals. Also emerging are corporate practices by psychiatrists, or physician organizations (POs). Successful PHOs and POs would presumably control the utilization of medical services and win patients, contracts, and shrinking revenues (Goldstein 1992; Sederer 1991).

A PHO or a PO is a physician-controlled corporation that distributes earnings to its physician members or shareholders on the basis of what surplus remains after all expenses are paid. The greater proportion of capitated or prospective payment (as opposed to fee-for-service) the group receives, the more at risk will be the compensation of its members. Simply put, what the group spends diminishes its salaries. What they save in administration and service delivery "drops to the bottom line" for distribution to the professional members. Psychiatrists (and other mental health professionals) managing care in PHOs will be rapidly sensitized to every purchase or expense. Their attention will be drawn to managing a practice—as employers and experts in how, when, and by whom care is rendered.

The movement toward PHOs and POs derives also from recent changes in managed care (Sederer and Bennett 1996). The micromanagement of benefits (demand reduction) is now being replaced by "supply side engineering," in which populations of patients are being managed by select clinician groups. Financial risk and exacting performance standards for access, satisfaction, and quality are among the criteria for the selection of clinician members (Epstein 1990; Sederer et al. 1995). PHOs and POs exemplify the way in which professionals are organizing themselves to be players in the new managed systems of care. Psychiatrists are discovering that unless they step into the role of employer, manager, or partner in a corporate group practice, their clinical and financial future may be adversely effected.

The primary task of those professionals governing and operating a physician organization will be practice management. Successful practice management will involve keeping costs below revenues, ensuring accessible services (see the next section for a discussion of quality), maintaining the satisfaction of patients, families, and any others involved in the purchase of care (e.g., insurers, managed care organizations), and meeting regulatory requirements (HCFA, JCAHO, IRS).

The primary tools of a psychiatrist-led professional practice will be its capital, budget, and monthly financial analyses; contracts with payers, members, and service partners; legal and ethical standards and procedures (Hinden and Elden 1990; Kopit and Lutes 1993); practice guidelines and related utilization management protocols; provider (member) selection and retention criteria; performance measures of access; and patient satisfaction surveys. Other chapters in this book offer more detailed examinations of these topics, each of which is crucial and warrants a lengthy discussion. Practice management is not a part of medical school or residency curricula. Most physicians have limited experience as employers or executives, and very few have any formal training. For many, these roles are a far cry from early career experience or ambitions. For some, such roles can seem a corruption of the values inherent in professional identify.

Cost containment and the corporatization of medical practice pose serious threats to the professionalism of psychiatry. The tenets of professionalism include the scientific method, expert opinion, autonomy, and ethics. Unless the professional paradigm is merged with accountability and affordability, however, the future of clinical practice will slip out of the hands of doctors. Our challenge is to prevent this from happening.

Psychiatrists as Leaders

The revolution in the financing and delivery of psychiatric services has ushered in a new epoch for psychiatry. There is comfort to be taken, however, in the history of psychiatry, which reveals its epochal nature. Modern psychiatry began with the introduction of "moral therapy" in the early 1800s. Humane treatment and the well-tended asylum guided our field throughout that century (and established the forerunner of organized American psychiatry through the work of a small group of superintendents of "insane asylums"). In time, a variety of economic and social forces conspired to diminish psychiatric services to custodial care (Rothman 1971; Sederer 1977). A second epoch then emerged, built on the techniques Freud advanced through his theory of the mind: namely, psychoanalysis and dynamic psychotherapy. American psychiatry was dominated by dynamic psychiatry through the first half of this century. After World War II, again inspired by new technologies (the introduction of new drugs such as lithium, neuroleptics, antidepressants, and anxiolytics, and new techniques such as brain imaging, epidemiology, and biostatistics), the epoch of biomedical psychiatry flowered. Psychiatry was increasingly medicalized, and the decade of the brain became inevitable.

Each epoch has had psychiatrists at its helm: Pinel, Esquirol, the Tukes, Rush, Earl from the moral era, Freud, Sullivan, Meyer, A. Adler, K. Menninger for the dynamic era, and many of our current leaders and contemporaries for the biomedicalization of psychiatry. And for each leader of national or international stature, many other leaders provided critical roles in every state, city, and psychiatric facility. The heat of today's health care crucible offers the energy to advance our profession. In this firestorm of health care financing, reform, and revolution lies the opportunity for psychiatric leadership.

Leadership will require that the field of psychiatry and its tens of thousands of practitioners carry forward a tradition of patient-oriented care, informed by empirical knowledge and human wisdom and shaped by the exigencies of the economics of medicine. The demands are substantial, but so are the potential rewards. Only through a leadership role will psychiatrists obtain the satisfaction essential to professional practice, the sense of achievement necessary for a life of initiative and industry, the financial security needed for equanimity, and the personal experience of integrity that derives from the just pursuit of the social good.

References

Annas GJ: Standard of Care: The Law of American Bioethics. New York, Oxford University Press, 1993

Appelbaum PS: Legal liability and managed care. Am Psychol, March 1993, pp 251–257

Baker LC, Cantor JC: Physician satisfaction under managed care. Health Aff (suppl):258–270, 1993

Berwick DM: Continuous improvement as an idea in health care. N Engl J Med 320:53–56, 1989

Brown LD: Who shall pay? Politics, money, and health care reform. Health Aff Spring 1994, p. 178

Donabedian A: Explorations in Quality Assurance and Monitoring, Vol 3. Ann Arbor, MI, Health Administration Press, 1985

Eisen SV, Grob MC, Dill DC: Outcome measurement: tapping the patient's perspective, in Psychiatric Treatment: Advances in Outcome Research. Edited by Mirin SM. Washington, DC, American Psychiatric Press, 1991

Enthoven AC: Health Plan: The Only Practical Solution to Soaring Health Costs. Reading, MA, Addison-Wesley, 1980

Enthoven AC: Why managed care has failed to contain costs. Health Aff 12:27–43, 1993

Epstein AM: The outcomes movement: will it get us where we want to go? N Engl J Med 323:266–270, 1990

Ernst & Young: Hospital physician integration: results of a national survey, 1993

Fein R: Medical Care, Medical Costs. Cambridge, MA, Harvard University Press, 1986

Fink PJ: Psychiatrists' roles in managed care programs. Hosp Community Psychiatry 44:723–724, 1993

Ginzberg E: Physician supply policies and health reform. JAMA 268: 3115–3118, 1992

Goldstein D: From Physician Bonding to Alliances: Building New Physician-Hospital Relationships. Washington, DC, Capitol Publications, 1992

Greco JP, Eisenberg JM: Changing physicians' practices. N Engl J Med 329:1271–1273, 1993

Hinden RA, Elden DL: Liability issues for managed care entities. Seton Hall Legislative Journal 14:1–63, 1990

Kahn A: Why incentive plans cannot work. Harvard Business Review, September–October 1993, pp 54–63

Kassirer JP: The use and abuse of practice profiles. N Engl J Med 330: 634–635, 1994

Katon W. Paper presented at the meeting of the American Association of Chairmen of Academic Departments, Seattle, WA, June 1993

Kessler LG, Cleary PD, Burke JD: Psychiatric disorders in primary care: results of a follow-up study. Arch Gen Psychiatry 42:583–587, 1985

Kopit, WG, Lutes ME: Legal issues and antitrust considerations in the establishment of credentialing and other selected criteria, in The Managed Health Care Handbook, 2nd Edition. Edited by Kongstvedt PR. Gaithersburg MD, Aspen, 1993

McCormick B: What price patient advocacy? American Medical Association News March 28, 1994, pp 1–6

McGlynn EA, Norquist GS, Wells KB, et al: Quality of care research in mental health: responding to the challenge. Inquiry 25:157–170, 1988

Mechanic D: From Advocacy to Allocation: The Evolving American Health Care System. New York, Free Press, 1986

Morreim EH: The new economics of medicine: special challenges for psychiatry. J Med Philos 15:97–119, 1990
Morreim EH: Economic disclosure and economic advocacy. J Leg Med 12:275–329, 1991
Narrow WE, Regier DA, Rae DS: Use of services by persons with mental and addictive disorders: findings from the NIMH epidemiologic catchment area program. Arch Gen Psychiatry 50: 95–107, 1933
Ormel J, Oldehinkel T, Brilman E, et al: Outcome of depression and anxiety in primary care. Arch Gen Psychiatry 50:759–766, 1993
Reames HR, Dunstone DC: Professional satisfaction of physicians. Arch Intern Med 149:1951–1956, 1989
Relman AS: Assessment and accountability: the third revolution in medical care. N Engl J Med 319:1220–1222, 1988
Rothman DJ: The Discovery of the Asylum. Boston, MA, Little, Brown, 1971
Schultz R, Girard C, Scheckler WE: Physician satisfaction in a managed care environment. J Fam Pract 3:298–304, 1992
Sederer LI: Moral therapy and the problem of morale. Am J Psychiatry 134:267–272, 1977
Sederer LI: Quality, costs and contracts, in Inpatient Psychiatry: Diagnosis and Treatment, 3rd Edition. Edited by Sederer LI. Baltimore, MD, Williams & Wilkins, 1991, pp 419–431
Sederer LI: Managed mental health care and professional compensation. Behav Sci Law 12:367–378, 1994
Sederer LI, Bennett MJ: Managed mental health care in the U.S.: a status report. Administration and Policy in Mental Health 23:289–306, 1996
Sederer LI, Randolph P, Jacobson G: Workshop on MPS members survey at the annual meeting of the American Psychiatric Association, Philadelphia, PA, May 1994
Sederer LI, Dickey B, Hermann R: The imperative of outcomes assessment in psychiatry. Am J Med Qual 10:127–132, 1995
Stoline A, Weiner JP: The New Medical Marketplace. Baltimore, MD, Johns Hopkins University Press, 1988
Thompson DF: Hospital ethics. Camb Q Healthc Ethics 3:203–215, 1992
Tischler G: Utilization management of mental health services by private third parties. Am J Psychiatry 147:467–473, 1990
Wells KB, Katon W, Rogers B, et al: The use of minor tranquilizers and antidepressant medications by depressed outpatients: results from the medical outcomes study. Am J Psychiatry 151:694–700, 1994

CHAPTER FOUR

Clinical Role of the Psychiatrist in Managed Care

Alan A. Axelson, M.D.

A widely quoted article in the January 1993 issue of the *New England Journal of Medicine* put psychiatrists at the top of the list of specialists that are in oversupply (Kronich 1993). Based on the number of psychiatrists per thousand covered live in health maintenance organizations, there is a surplus of more than 70%. When I mentioned this in a presentation, a member of the audience appropriately asked, "If there is such a surplus of psychiatrists, why is it that we can't find any psychiatrists to work with us in our programs?"

We are certainly in a confusing period when experts on one hand say that there is a great surplus of psychiatrists, and other experts indicate that only a minority of individuals are receiving adequate treatment for psychiatric illness. To be sure, there is considerable anxiety about the economic future for psychiatrists. When you listen carefully, the issue is not whether there will be work available at reasonable compensation for treatment of patients with psychiatric illness; rather, it is concern over the clinical role, the practice setting, scope of responsibility, and, particularly, autonomy for those physicians who are established in the practice of psychiatry.

This tension about the clinical role of the psychiatrist in managed care is the manifest or at least latent concern when psychiatrists gather in groups for discussion. It was the formal topic of the all-day Traverse City conference on the role of child psychiatrists in systems of care sponsored by the Robert Wood Johnson Foundation (Washington Business Group on Health 1994). It is also a major agenda item when the Work Group on Managed Care of the American Academy of Child and Adolescent Psychiatry meets twice yearly with the Academy's Assembly of Regional Organizations. The process of rapid change and reorganization in systems of psychiatric care is chronicled by one representative after another. The Assembly of the American Psychiatric Association regularly produces a number of action papers directed toward stemming the tide of change. These are discussed in the APA Managed Care Committee as well as other components of the APA. As one listens to the discussion, it is important to differentiate the voices resisting change from those trying to shape change.

It appears, at least from informal discussions, that the psychiatrists who feel most vulnerable are those in solo psychotherapy practice with a fee-for-service patient group supported by insurance. Not only is the rate per session, frequency of treatment, and duration of treatment being challenged, but there are a large number of administrative complications. Having to frequently seek approval and complete unique documentation for a number of different managed care companies is making solo-type practice almost untenable. The opportunity to practice in inpatient settings devoted to the long-term active treatment of serious psychiatric illness has been substantially curtailed as days of stay in inpatient settings are often now in the single digits. For a time psychiatrists practicing at academic institutions had some insulation from the impact of these changes. Now these programs are feeling the impact of economic forces, and they, too, are dramatically reengineering their programs and asking psychiatrists to take on different clinical roles. For a while, the concerns were considered as something that might happen or were seen as events occurring someplace else. Now, major program changes precipitated by managed care are occurring in academic programs in nearly every metropolitan community.

What is going on is the rapid restructuring of health care. It is now being reshaped more by forces of the marketplace than by individual practice patterns and the recommendation of the attending physician.

To deal with the powerful trends that threaten our capacity to treat our patients, we need to be proactive in clearly establishing our clinical roles. Defensive actions (e.g., critical broadsides against managed care or nonproductive communications with managed care psychiatrists) dissipate resources and divert the psychiatric community from the goal of establishing an effective behavioral health care system for the future. The forces of non-productive market-oriented behavioral health care having impact and popularity today vary in strength and empirical support. It is time to establish positions of confidence and push back in our interactions with managed care companies to maintain quality care for our patients. Well-established scientific principles and economic fundamentals are now being challenged by market expediency. We must effectively assert our clinical role, based not on what is traditional but on what is effective and what accomplishes the goal of improving the health status of the community within the bounds of prudent use of available resources. We must participate in this process of change with civility and integrity, and we must work to hold other participants in this process to the same standards.

Conceptually, the best managed care is about a systems approach: the interaction between patient needs and health care resources, guided by principles of quality management and benchmarks for health outcome. Using a systems approach, the various components of the service system needed by the patient are integrated to form a continuum that brings to bear the appropriate resources at the appropriate time.

What is the role of the psychiatrist clinician confronting the suffering patient, the needy family, effective but sometimes expensive treatments, idealistic concepts of smoothly functioning integrated systems, and the realities of a business-oriented marketplace that makes cost control a first priority? First and foremost, it is to be with the patient and make some sense of the various factors in the patient's situation, indicating strengths and weaknesses, and identifying opportunities for improvement. The patient, and at times his or her family, are suffering the stress and disorganization of a psychiatric illness. The psychiatrist must put that experience in a framework that supports constructive action and then work with available treatment resources to implement that action. Other mental health professionals can often be very effective as well in this process, but the broader training of the psychiatrist in biological, psychological, and social factors, as well as the training and socialization as a physician with all its continuing responsibilities for education and licensure, makes psychiatrists critical members of the teams responsible for the treatment of patients with psychiatric illness.

Crisis Assessment

The psychiatrist must play a central role in the organization, management, and operation of the teams of professionals responsible for managing emergency response and triage systems. When patients or families are identified as being involved in high-stress or high-risk situations, the most experienced and broadly trained staff can responsibly initiate the application of only those resources necessary to deal with the situation. The psychiatrist must not only appropriately assess the situation but also engender the confidence of the patient and family that the recommended course of action is the one that is necessary and deserves their cooperation and support. The psychiatrist presents treatment alternatives and should be able to describe and assist in decision making that balances both clinical and economic factors. Decisions made in the first hours of crisis often determine its outcome from both a clinical and economic perspective. Today's climate of developing cost-effective care puts the psychiatrist on the front line in evaluating a patient whose clinical condition indicates the possibility that inpatient psychiatric treatment may be necessary. This may be supporting a mobile crisis team as in a psychiatric emergency department.

Management of High-Risk Patients

The second very clear role for the psychiatrist is the management of high-risk patients. Fortunately, many crises are resolved quickly with patients stabilizing and being managed in lower intensity treatment settings. When the evaluation of the patient indicates persistent risk of self-destructive behavior or violence related to the presence of mental illness, our clinical systems and our legal system still expect that the professional with the broadest training—the psychiatrist—will have the ultimate responsibility for the management of these patients. Managed care has heightened the importance of this role by requiring that patients be treated in less intensive settings. No longer does the possibility of threatening behavior justify the application of secure treatment; the patients must demonstrate the clear risk of danger. The profession should work with reputable managed care companies to support psychiatrists' responsible involvement in these decisions.

Team Involvement

Generally, psychiatrists working in a managed care environment practice most efficiently when they are members of a team. This is in recognition of the fact that the implementation of some aspects of our treatment plans do not require a person with the comprehensive training of a psychiatrist. In fact, to the extent that the therapeutic intervention requires a highly specialized skill, there may be others who, because of training and experience, exceed the psychiatrist's capability as a group therapist, a family therapist, or one skilled in cognitive therapy or interactive therapy.

The Traverse City Conference on Child and Adolescent Psychiatrists' Roles in Systems of Care (Washington Business Group on Health 1994) broadly supported the idea that the psychiatrist's involvement as part of a team was highly prized and in great demand by consumers and other professionals. In this role of essential team member, psychiatrists are called upon to be the integrator of biopsychosocial information in highly complex situations. They are also asked to be brokers of treatment services from outside sources, particularly those required from resistant and difficult providers. As part of teams, psychiatrists supervise, teach, consult, and collaborate. They are often responsible for the integration of the team's activities with other medical services. As a team member, the psychiatrist is often responsible for dealing with other psychiatrists and physicians in the process of transition as the patient moves from high- to lower-intensity treatment or the reverse. In the time- and resource-pressured world of managed care, these transitions are critical. Psychiatrists often bear the responsibility of deciding when the transition is appropriate. At times, they must challenge the authorization of the managed care company reviewer who applies the company's criteria from a distance and may not be sensitive to the various factors that must be weighed when deciding to discharge from the hospital to an outpatient or partial hospital-treatment setting.

Although psychiatrists working in inpatient or partial hospital-treatment programs are comfortable working as members of teams, many psychiatrists in outpatient practice still see this as a solo endeavor. This is in contrast to our other medical colleagues who, even when in solo practice, are assisted by nurses or other office personnel. Even though there are still a number of patients who are effectively and efficiently treated by a psychiatrist in solo office practice, the range of effective treatments available today for patients and the complexity of the administrative support systems required by the managed care environment encourage the development of teamwork in outpatient settings, as well as in the higher intensity partial hospital and inpatient programs. The demands for accessibility and the range of the patient's needs from brief counseling to long-term outpatient management of serious psychiatric illnesses support the organization of group practices where psychiatrists work with other mental health professionals to offer a comprehensive range of outpatient services. The psychiatrist's role in these outpatient settings is often determined by who has taken the initiative to organize the group and therefore exercises management control. In groups that are physician organized and led, psychiatrists may determine the composition of the group and the roles of professionals who participate. Some contracts between group practices and managed care companies give wide latitude to the group in terms of assignment of the clinical cases. These delegated management arrangements allow the professionals in the group to determine their own policies regarding the involvement of the psychiatrist in assessment, treatment planning, and treatment implementation. When psychologists, social workers, or other professionals have taken the initiative to organize a group practice, the psychiatrist's role may be more limited, focusing on high-risk patients and those requiring pharmacologic intervention. The standards set forth by the Council of Behavioral Group Practices of the Institute for Behavioral Healthcare[1] require that, to be a member, the group practice must have psychiatrists as an

---

[1] Led by Michael A. Freeman, M.D., the Institute for Behavioral Healthcare is a non-profit corporation that promotes development, quality, and value in behavioral healthcare through the sponsorship of multidisciplinary conferences and educational programs. They are located at 1110 Mar West Street, Suite E, Tiburon, CA 94920.

integral part of the group rather than being involved only as a consultant or in some other limited role. In the group practice model, the psychiatrist/mental health professional teams can manage patients together, each complementing the other's skills. These skill sets may be in specific types of psychotherapy, working with patients with specialized problems such as posttraumatic stress disorder or anorexia, the coordination of care with schools and different agencies, or the management of psychotherapeutic medications and the psychiatric aspects of medical illnesses. In this outpatient group-practice teamwork, a collegial relationship facilitates patient care, bringing in the psychiatrist to work out a complex diagnosis, deal with an anxious or resistant family, or provide the physician authority that is important when confirming the diagnosis of a serious psychiatric illness. In the group practice model, managed care companies are often more confident that there can be alignment between the principles of the managed care company and those of the clinical program, allowing for decrease in the level of managed care intrusion into the treatment process.

Solo Practice

In communities where there is a high penetration of managed care, is there a role for the psychiatrist in solo outpatient practice? Certainly those psychiatrists who practice in areas where there is a relative scarcity or those who have well-known local reputations or special skills in dealing with specific populations will continue to be in demand. It is likely, however, that they must be part of networks or provider panels and therefore be responsive to the requirements of those systems. Working with several responsive managed care systems that provide a significant volume of patients in one's practice is a manageable task. Dealing with 10 or 12 different companies, each with different forms, utilization criteria, appeals processes, and expectations in terms of responsiveness will be an overwhelming task that requires a good deal of administrative time, apart from dealing with the clinical needs of patients. Often, managed care companies value the psychiatrist's psychopharmacologic skills and will be reluctant to refer patients who need only psychotherapy. Because of these established patterns, being a solo practice psychiatrist in a managed care environment will be very difficult unless there are substantial changes in the way that managed care companies discharge their responsibilities.

Psychopharmacologic Management

One role that will make the list of "five probable roles for a psychiatrist when there is 100% enrollment in managed care" is responsibility for the management of psychotropic medications. There is certainly ample evidence that medication plays a prominent role in the effective treatment of many serious psychiatric illnesses. Applying our diagnostic acumen, our understanding of neurobiology, and, we hope, our up-to-date knowledge of the available psychotropic medications, we expect that their applications, side effects, and management will provide a secure position for the psychiatrists who are comfortable in this role. There are factors, however, that unless assertively addressed make even this role insecure. If our practice settings and geographic locations are such that a minority of those with a psychiatric illness who can benefit from these services actually receive the services of psychiatrists, there will be considerable pressure to vest the management of medications in the hands of the nonspecialist primary care physician and midlevel practitioners (i.e., nurse practitioners and physician's assistants, or even non-medically trained professionals such as psychologists). For many categories of psychotropic medications, nonpsychiatrist physicians are responsible for the majority of the prescriptions. The process of diagnosis, treatment, and continued management can be trivialized by a managed care company allowing four, brief, 10-minute visits per year for the management of a stable bipolar patient on lithium. The administrative process is so cumbersome and the return so small that the psychiatrist often accepts the inadequate authorization for each visit and provides the necessary time for a visit without challenging the managed care company's time allocation. As more data accumulate regarding the synergistic interaction of psychotherapeutically based patient management and psychotropic medication management, sophisticated care management systems will vest in the psychiatrist, the combined responsibility of diagnosis and ongoing treatment for patients with psychiatric illnesses who require psychotropic medication. Patients are likely to benefit from this combination, and psychiatrists will experience greater professional satisfaction. To do this, however, we must embrace this role, evaluate the various parameters related to its advocacy and availability, and negotiate for compensation consistent with the value of the service. We need to determine when it is appropriate to share responsibility with our physician colleagues in primary care and in what settings it is appropriate for nurse practitioners or physician's assistants to participate in the process of ongoing medication monitoring. Without assertive steps in these directions, we will miss an opportunity to secure for psychiatrists an important essential role.

Outpatient Consultation With Primary Care

Some psychiatrists have well-established roles as consultants to general practitioners, internists, and other medical specialists. Often these patterns are based on long-term personal relationships, medical staff memberships, or participation in a multispecialty group practice, medical center, or academic program. Often the teamwork between psychiatric and medical colleagues has been very productive and satisfying for both the professionals and the patients. Despite these positive factors, it is unlikely that even these close professional relationships will be protected from the changes of managed care. The establishment of limited preferred provider networks often do not account for established consultation patterns. Primary care physicians must use consultants that are in the preferred provider organization (PPO) network, and patients may be encouraged to use direct access rather than going through their primary care physician. It has generally been the experience of network-based health maintenance organizations (HMOs) that informal referral relationships are not sufficient to take care of the urgent and complex psychiatric and substance abuse treatment needs of a large population of people. Assurances regarding access and consistency of treatment have led many of them to carve out behavioral health services into separately managed units. When the

HMO/PPO contracts have a point-of-service option, the referring physician can encourage the patient to utilize the psychiatrist with whom he or she has the long-standing referral relationship. In most cases, however, it will be the carve out that determines the referral.

The physician hospital organizations—business entities joining the resources and interests of hospitals and their medical staffs—are too new to evaluate what impact they will have on consultation relationships between psychiatrists and primary care and specialist physicians, but there are some common issues that should prompt us to develop methods of enhancing our contribution to these medical systems. The common element is that services provided to populations of people will be more carefully tracked and evaluated. The number of psychiatric consultations by one primary care physician may be contrasted with those by another, and legitimate questions will be asked about the appropriate use of psychiatric consultation. The considerable literature on the decreased utilization of medical services when psychiatric services are available to patients who present with physical symptoms may have strong practical application. This will be accomplished only if the profession as a whole and the psychiatrists who work individually in these systems take the initiative to highlight these benefits and truly make them available to patients and referring physicians.

Other mental health disciplines recognize the need for behavioral health services to provide close support for primary care physicians. Primary care physicians may directly hire social workers and psychologists to work within their offices with the primary care physicians providing psychotropic medications. Although this may enhance the sensitivity to psychosocial issues, it will not bring integrated behavioral health services to the primary care setting. Outreach teams of mental health professionals supported by psychiatrists that are part of integrated services' networks can provide the full range of psychiatric support to the primary care setting that is necessary for true integrated systems. Mental health professionals available on a part-time basis in the primary care physician's office can provide easily accessible services. When psychiatric consultation is appropriate, they can facilitate the process and integrate recommendations into the patient's primary care.

Systems-Oriented Practice

Another key way to enhance patient care and retain an essential role in providing that care is to thoroughly understand and apply the principles of quality management to our clinical practice. Through the American Academy of Child and Adolescent Psychiatry, the American Psychiatric Association, and academic, research, and governmental organizations, psychiatrists as a group are taking significant steps forward in establishing scientifically based treatment guidelines that may significantly increase the quality of care and reduce the cost of care. The key to this process, of course, is broad participation in the development and continued evolution and consistent application of these guidelines in clinical settings. This cannot be left to those psychiatrists who are in administrative positions but must be a priority for the psychiatrist involved in daily patient care. The extensive literature related to quality improvement and the applications of practice guidelines should become part of our processes of training and continuing education. James (1993) provides an excellent review of the process of the development and application of practice guidelines. By taking a leadership role in the development of treatment guidelines for psychiatric patients and insisting on their application in clinical practice, we can develop systems that provide optimal care for patients.

Roles to Avoid

There are several roles that psychiatrists must avoid. The first is assuming clinical responsibility without sufficient clinical support. Managed care pushes the envelope, asking psychiatrists to treat patients using fewer resources. Psychiatrists must assess the available system of care and the part they can play in that system and then determine whether they can ethically take responsibility for their role in the care of the patient. There is no question that once the psychiatrist has entered into a contract with a patient for care, he or she has a responsibility to fulfill that contract. When the psychiatrist deals with patients through managed care contracts, the patient will need to clearly understand the boundaries of the psychiatrist's services and the role the psychiatrist plays in assisting the patient in obtaining needed services.

In the first encounter with the patient, the psychiatrist should clearly establish the boundaries of his or her role. It may be limited to providing an assessment or consultation regarding the patient's current status and treatment needs. Once the psychiatrist has moved past the assessment and entered into a contract for treatment, a continuing responsibility exists that must be carefully transferred if the psychiatrist is no longer able to fulfill the treatment contract. Some managed care organizations (MCOs) do not adequately appreciate and support this medical responsibility and therefore make functioning within them difficult, if not untenable. A clear example of this problem is the MCO that severely restricts the duration of inpatient care without adequately supporting alternative treatment such as partial hospitalization, intensive residential treatment, and intensive outpatient treatment. Clinically, this makes as much sense as the denial of coverage for outpatient surgery as an alternative to inpatient surgery or the discharge of mothers 36 hours after delivering without in-home nursing and high-intensity obstetric and pediatric support. Benefit limits have long been used to control utilization of psychiatric treatment services. The failure to implement a broader benefit for alternative and outpatient services while using the considerable power of managed care review to limit inpatient services puts the patient and the psychiatrist in a dangerous clinical position where hospitalization is no longer justified but partial hospital or intensive outpatient services are not available. Enlightened benefits consultants and national managed care companies recognize this and have encouraged larger companies to develop benefit plans to cover partial hospitalization and outpatient treatment as an alternative to inpatient stays. As the principles of managed care have been applied more broadly and involve smaller companies, partial hospitalization is viewed as an additional benefit rather than an appropriate alternative to inpatient treatment. The insurer and the managed care company take the position that they are unable to dictate a change in benefits to the business owners that actually determine the scope of their self-insured plans. When faced with this dilemma, the psychiatrist must actively advocate for his or her patient to receive a higher level of care if alternative treatments are not practically available.

Another common practice that should be resisted is the discontinuity that occurs when there is no real relationship between the psychiatrist who manages medication and the clinician who actually conducts the psychotherapy and case management. It is my experience that master's and Ph.D.-level professionals, when part of a team that includes a psychiatrist, can effectively provide case management, psychotherapy, and supportive services to patients with serious psychiatric illness who require medication. This effective teamwork occurs when the mental health professional and the psychiatrist have a high degree of mutual trust and communication. When the managed care company's network contains a number of solo practice mental health practitioners who do not have relationships with psychiatrists, the psychiatrist may be used only as a consultant for medication. In these situations, the managed care companies fail to recognize and financially support the amount of communication that must go on between the therapist and the psychiatrist. They seem to deny the fact that the psychiatrist cannot have a narrow responsibility for the patient. Having become part of the ongoing treatment process, the psychiatrist can be considered as sharing responsibility for the actions of the psychotherapist.

The heart of managed care is about contracts—contracts between the psychiatrist and the managed care company, contracts between the psychiatrist and the patient, and contracts between the insurer and the patient through the managed care company. Contracts are meant to promote an understanding of responsibilities, rewards, and penalties, establishing systems of care. Psychiatrists, as individuals and as groups, must clearly understand the nature of these contractual relationships and be prepared to either live up to the contract, modify it, or reject it. Working as a clinician in an environment with managed care requires a rethinking of our paradigm of treatment and a careful application of our clinical expertise and professional standards. We must be prepared to shape this system assertively as we deal with individual patients, groups of patients, and systems as a whole. I believe this is best done if we recognize the positive values of care management and understand why it has been successful in the marketplace of health care. Only then can we effectively address its inefficiencies, excesses, improper implementation, and unprincipled applications. No matter what the global system, the crucial clinical encounter is the interaction between the patient and psychiatrist, understanding the nature of the patient's suffering and mental illness and implementing plans to improve the patient's health. Managed care becomes one of the parameters that affects this treatment process. By keeping our eye on its manifest and latent implications, we can maintain our responsibility to our patients and our professional integrity.

Managed care developed because of unacceptable variations in care and associated high costs. The clinical role for psychiatrists in a managed care environment is going to depend on the nature of that environment. James sums up the situation: "For the next generation of American health care systems, success will depend on the ability of health care leaders to create a culture of cooperation among all members of the health care team. Those leaders will not manage physicians. Instead, they will organize clinicians and then supply them with the necessary tools so that physicians can manage themselves and the health care processes they oversee. In creating that collaborative culture, it is obviously far more important how health care leaders implement practice guidelines, than the particular set of guidelines they used to initiate implementation" (James 1993).

As clinicians, we must participate in that culture of cooperation and continuous quality improvement. If we do so, we will have satisfying professional roles, and our patients will benefit from scientifically based treatment.

References

James, BC: Implementing practice guidelines through clinical quality improvement. Front Health Serv Manage 10:1, 1993

Kronich R, Goodman DC, Wennberg E, et al: The marketplace in healthcare reform: the demographic limitations of managed competition. N Engl J Med 328:148–152, 1993

Washington Business Group on Health and The Robert Wood Johnson Foundation: Synopsis of the June 18–19, 1994, conference at the Grand Traverse Village, Traverse City, MI

CHAPTER FIVE

Administrative Psychiatry and Managed Care: Advances and Opportunities

Ronald D. Geraty, M.D.

Over the last 20 years, marked changes in attitudes and conditions within the social and health care environments have intensified the financial significance of mental health care benefits. The broadening of societal awareness of mental health and substance abuse problems, the reduction in the traditional stigma attached to psychiatric treatment, the growth in the number of private psychiatric hospital beds, and the proliferation of state-mandated mental health care benefit coverage laws were developments that served to increase the degree to which treatment services were utilized.

As utilization grew, the aggregate cost of care expanded to unprecedented levels. And those groups paying for mental health benefits, particularly employer sponsors of relatively benefit-rich health plans, encountered the considerable challenge of maintaining coverages in the face of skyrocketing costs. When medical-surgical utilization review organizations were unable to respond effectively to the financial and operational complexities of the mental health care system, managed behavioral health care specialty companies emerged.

The continuing success of managed behavioral health care firms has been grounded in the ability to reduce costs significantly while improving access to care and demonstrating quality (Geraty 1994). To date, managed behavioral health care has distinguished itself by its effective management of care delivery and not by transforming the basic elements of treatment, namely, the initial diagnostic assessment and treatment plan. Through individualized case management techniques applied within multidisciplinary specialty networks using a full continuum of treatment settings, the needs of patients and payers have been met.

In addressing payer demands and managing the imperatives of the market, managed behavioral health care companies have changed the traditional methods of care delivery and altered the professional milieu. The presence of large multidisciplinary provider networks has contributed to the continuing lively debate over the appropriate roles to be played by the various mental health professions. The managed behavioral health care industry fully recognizes the primary clinical role that the psychiatric profession must perform in any system that intends to serve the full spectrum of treatment needs that arises in a broad patient population. And beyond strictly clinical functions, evolving managed behavioral health care systems are expanding the administrative opportunities for psychiatrists who have the breadth of training and experience typified by the profession.

Current developments in *managed* behavioral health care will stretch the scope of psychiatry and further broaden a professional vision that encompasses the full potential of delivery systems that will inevitably advance the effectiveness and value of psychiatric treatment. Clinical progress will depend on the skill of psychiatric clinicians and administrators who are able to direct the delivery of care in a manner that contributes to and employs an exponentially expanding knowledge base.

Health Care Reform and Market Forces

Health care reform, in whatever forms it may take, will have a major effect on the provision of care. Expanding access to mental illness and substance abuse treatment is a key objective in all viable reform plans under consideration, and the extension of public coverage programs is expected to play an important role in that expansion. Not only will millions of currently uninsured persons gain access to treatment, but it is likely that those patient populations now insured through Medicare and Medicaid programs will be aided by more comprehensive mental benefit packages.

Moreover, health care reform will almost certainly result in the eventual establishment of some form of national health care quality standards. New yardsticks for measuring the effectiveness of and patient satisfaction with mental health care will affect therapeutic practice.

It is no coincidence that these expected effects of health care reform mirror present trends in the managed health care industry since the basic goals of reform—cost-effectiveness, improved access, and high-quality care—have been anticipated by market forces and are already being served by managed behavioral health care.

Not surprisingly, public mental health programs, in great need of systematic solutions to cost, access, and quality concerns, represent the most important emerging market for managed behavioral health care. Although much work remains to be done, industry innovations have proven successful in helping to improve services under public programs.

In both the public and private sectors, the efficacy of behavioral health systems is being gauged by increasingly sophisticated standards. Although managed behavioral health care has demonstrated very successfully the ability to produce cost savings, improve access, and maintain quality, demands for more advanced measures of value are spurring managed behavioral health care toward the new arena of demonstrable competitive worth—improved treatment outcomes (Marques et al. 1994). Positive outcomes are the strongest indicator of high-quality treatment, and the formation of new treatment delivery systems that integrate the operational and clinical elements crucial to ensuring optimal treatment outcomes is required.

The further refinement of delivery systems administration will entail the enlistment of all the experience and versatility that the psychiatric profession can bring to bear in managing complex public patient populations and achieving improved outcomes. The exercise of that professionalism within new integrated delivery systems adapted to the necessities of the mental health care environment will provide the most productive opportunities in the future of psychiatry.

Psychiatrists, Integrated Delivery Systems, and Change

Delivery systems can no longer comfortably maintain a conceptual boundary between the roles of the psychiatrist/practitioner and the mental health administrator. The need to continually inform and improve the delivery of care through the collection and channeling of treatment data has become more apparent than ever before. Change has become the rule, and the daily interplay between administrator and practitioner will be the fundamental driver of positive change.

> It has forced a new recognition that the psychiatrist must become systems-relevant as well as patient-focused, and that the manager/administrator . . . must become clinically sophisticated about the therapeutic requirements of the patients that system is treating.
>
> For both has come the necessity that their roles evolve into larger and more broadly responsible sets of functions, both in terms of devising the steps and strategies that will enable necessary adaptive changes, and to insure that they occur. Even more critically, both the administrator and the psychiatrist-manager have had to acquire the skills of an anticipatory planner as a precondition to knowing just which changes to make. (Menninger 1993)

Although the early cost containment successes of managed care certainly addressed the crucial financial concern of the time, that narrower management focus is now outdated. The failure of some less sophisticated managed care systems to broaden and better coordinate the administrative and caregiving functions had been earlier identified from a physician's point of view as a primary reason for a lack of innovation (Berenson 1991). In spite of considerable successes, a perceived overemphasis on administrative efficiency was seen as undermining more ambitious efforts to improve the long-term effectiveness of the delivery system.

Now that quality management is taking center stage in the evolution of managed behavioral care, a management revolution in mental health care delivery will require a renewed commitment to clinical and administrative medical professionalism. Psychiatrists are the most appropriate managers for the clinical delivery of care. However, although psychotherapeutic treatment has been shown to correlate with an improved mental state, standards for intensity, length, and appropriateness of treatment methods for various conditions have not been clearly established (Gottlieb 1989). Clarification of such treatment performance standards is needed to form sounder measures of clinical quality and value, but improving quality of care and patient outcomes will require sophisticated systems for collecting comprehensive data on patient populations, service costs, patient satisfaction, and treatment settings, modalities, and efficacy.

Integrated behavioral health care systems are emerging as the answer to the growing need to systematize and harmonize clinical and administrative objectives. Such systems will integrate the full array of financial, operational, and clinical functions into one delivery organization. Integrating the assumption of financial risk for cost of care with the delivery of services for regional populations will be the basis for creating value. Organizing facilities, provider networks, and corporate operations into one design that encompasses prevention, wellness, and treatment will become the method of improving the mental health of diverse patient populations.

The movement toward integrated behavioral health care systems is evidenced by three current trends in the behavioral health industry (Bengen-Seltzer 1994a). First, managed care organizations are becoming involved in a higher level of horizontal and vertical integration activity. The related merger and acquisition trend is an indication of the market's desire for higher quality care and more refined cost savings measures through consolidated provider and manager efforts in care delivery.

Second, providers are expanding service offerings to complement managed care organization efforts to perfect the comprehensiveness of the continuum of care. Newly developing provider services and products include the following (Bengen-Seltzer 1994a):

- Twenty-three-hour holding beds
- Crisis stabilization units
- Mobile evaluation teams
- In-home crisis stabilization and treatment
- Group home services
- Triaging and referral services

Finally, there is an increasing overlap between the roles and functions of providers and managed care organizations. Through partnering relationships, behavioral health providers are moving to full risk-sharing roles in working with managed care organizations. As a result, providers of care must necessarily become deliverers of value as determined by the best quality of care at the lowest possible cost. Provider risk assumption is coming in the form of per episode fee arrangements and capitation payments. The advantages of these full-risk agreements include a clearer affirmation of provider treatment decision autonomy, elimination of certain provider and managed care organization utilization review complexities, and the abatement of detailed patient care delivery management by the managed care organization (Bengen-Seltzer 1994b). Further, through the larger patient volumes of these systems, economies of scale will be achieved.

However, risk assumption by providers requires enhanced administrative capabilities in the management of care and risk. Managing risk calls for well-developed administrative skills in finance, actuarial, and information systems. In addition, there is a heightened need for more sophisticated provider utilization management and effective processing and use of treatment outcome data. These greater administrative requirements have promoted much closer linkages between providers and managed care organizations in integrating the effective delivery of care.

The coordination of the full continuum of behavioral care—inpatient, respite, residential, partial hospital, intensive outpatient, in-home, and outpatient—will require new levels of cooperation and collegiality. And the need to better coordinate the provision of behavioral care with general medical practitioners must also be served. Enhanced provider accountability for quality and value will be essential, as will be rewards for efficiency and quality. The creation and application of methods to address the requisites of new integrated behavioral health care delivery systems will yield a panoply of new opportunities for psychiatrists and psychiatric institutions.

Administrative Psychiatry Within Integrated Delivery

The results of a study of over 19,000 psychiatrists surveyed during 1988–1989 indicated that psychiatrists as a group spent approximately

12% of their time on administrative activities (Dorwart et al. 1992). As of January 1, 1993, out of a total of 41,794 psychiatrists (including child and adolescent psychiatrists) in the United States, 2,029 were engaged primarily in administration (Physician Characteristics and Distribution in the U.S. 1994). With the expanding overlap in roles of providers and managers of care becoming even more pronounced in integrated systems, psychiatrists will serve the profession well by mastering a broader range of administrative skills. As stated in a general medical context, "[i]nstead of confronting the dictates of managers, physicians should become managers" (Berenson 1994). Psychiatrists are the appropriate managers for integrated behavioral health care delivery.

> It is up to medical professionals, to the extent they wish to claim the prerogative of professionals to be self-managing, to put the house of medicine in order. The responsibilities of professionalism need to be expanded beyond the bounds of individual technical competence to include an ecumenical responsibility for institutional performance, the profession's clinical practices, and the health system, including objective assessments and accountability for continuous improvement. (Etheredge and Jones 1991)

Integrated behavioral delivery systems now compose the most appropriate arena for accomplishing needed improvements, and professional resistance to this progression in the managed care environment is ill advised. The proposition that psychiatrists can well play a major role in shaping these systems is supported by practical experience. Feedback on utilization patterns are most effective when clinical leadership is involved in and supportive of such communications. It has also been shown that physician participation in the development of cost-saving programs in organized health care settings improves the success of such programs significantly (Gottlieb 1989). Both the breadth and depth of training and experience of psychiatrists makes them uniquely suited to administer behavioral health care systems.

Moreover, the anticipated "reintegration" of behavioral care systems with the general medical system is further reason for the prominent role of psychiatrists in the integrated delivery system. Specifically, managed behavioral health care systems are "carving" their management capabilities into the general medical health system in order to optimize the behavioral treatment efforts of primary care physicians (PCPs). It is estimated that 60% of behavioral health care is provided by PCPs (Marques et al. 1994). Carving-in fosters a higher degree of coordinated effort between managed behavioral and general medical health care delivery. On the clinical side, increased psychiatric consultation-liaison and on-site response activities will create a deeper need for systemic participation by psychiatrists. Administratively, the obvious bonds of professional collegiality and shared training emphasize the critical role for psychiatrists to play in managing an efficient flow of communication in working with PCPs to advance the effectiveness and outcome of overall behavioral health delivery. In this manner, PCP communications and education programs will promote more appropriate and timely behavioral treatment.

One must not ignore the fact that, during the early stages of managed behavioral health care, many psychiatrists have voiced great concerns about the perceived threat of cost-saving measures impinging on their clinical and ethical judgment. Utilization review and care delivery criteria have posed previously unencountered decision-making complexities. In treating patients, physicians embrace the values of autonomy, beneficence, and justice (Kane 1988; Povar 1988). These principles require the physician to maximize the right of patients to make decisions about their own lives (autonomy), act in the best interests of patients (beneficence), and make fair decisions for patients (justice). Yet, far from practicing in a vacuum, physicians have had to balance professional principles with a responsibility to the values of society at large. All corners of society have clamored for answers to runaway health care costs, and managed care delivery has been the one mechanism that has worked to effect responsible, value-balanced solutions. Administrative psychiatrists have played a major part in addressing the many clinical, ethical, and resource-allocation issues that have arisen, for it is the physician who retains ultimate responsibility for the delivery of care. In fact, a number of managed behavioral health care companies (American PsychManagement, Assured Health Systems, BenesYs, Preferred Health, TAO, and others) were founded by psychiatrists whose vision encompassed the administrative potential of accommodating both socioeconomic imperatives and time-honored canons of medical practice.

More importantly, we are now entering a new era in which the principles concerning patient autonomy, patient interests, and provider treatment decisions will find their greatest servant in managed behavioral health care systems. By virtue of the comprehensive clinical and operational databases of integrated behavioral health care systems, outcomes management will provide the learning and applications necessary to better inform patient choices and advance the efforts—of both psychiatrists and general medical practitioners alike—to achieve higher quality in their medical practice. The outcomes data revolution will afford the ability to assess and refine professional performance in unprecedented detail. It is here that psychiatrist-managers will play a crucial role. "Physicians are the best judges of other physicians' performance. Professional norms will always be the largest influence on medical practice" (White 1993). In managing an expanded realm of quality and outcomes management, administrative psychiatry will be the guiding hand in reaching new standards of progress.

Quality and Outcomes: Managing the Opportunity

It can be said of any discipline that the complete perfection of the science will quickly reduce the professional practice to the level of a commodity. In other words, if the psychiatric profession were to perfect all aspects of applied therapeutic methods and gain the ability to produce an optimal treatment outcome in every case of mental illness, the need for professional judgment would be obviated, and a therapeutic "cookbook" could replace the psychiatrist. However, given the long and winding road of outcome research that lies ahead of us, we know there is little need to fear impending obsolescence. Yet, there is no room for complacency. Rather, the psychiatric profession would do well to further embrace the opportunities presented by the management revolution taking place within integrated managed behavioral health care systems.

As previously mentioned, treatment quality measured in terms of positive outcomes will become a prime means of assessing the value of behavioral health care delivery. The managed behavioral health care industry is well positioned to contribute greatly to the overall advancement of outcomes management. Because of experience with hundreds of thousands of treatment episodes in the full continuum of treatment settings and under the widest variety of both public and private health benefit plans, managed behavioral health care has the expertise and information base necessary to timely progress in outcomes management (Marques et al. 1994). Industry trade associations and consumer groups have committed to advancing data collection, measurement, and reporting for further improving care delivery quality. In addition, under the aegis of the Center for Mental Health Services, the Evaluation Center at the Human Services Research Institute is working to foster the transition to management by outcomes and standards. Such management will be accomplished by the following (Mental Health Weekly 1994):

- Classifying conditions
- Estimating outcomes and costs
- Measuring societal preferences for outcomes
- Allocating resources based on available data and budget considerations

Integrated behavioral health care systems will have the mechanisms and administrative capacity to correct those factors that in the past have curtailed advancements in outcomes improvement. Progress has been made in elemental outcomes measurement (Caton and Gralnick 1987; Chandler et al. 1996; Crits-Christoph 1992; Renz et al. 1995). The focus is now turning to issues pertaining to specific appropriate treatment for specific disorders. The study of these questions involves innumerable variant combinations concerning treatment modality, setting, and intensity; length of treatment; timing of treatment intervention; and coordination of multidisciplinary provider functions. The data demands of such research present a formidable challenge. State-of-the-art information systems will play an integral part in the management of databases configured to the unexampled complexities of future outcome measurement (Sperry et al. 1996).

Furthermore, effective communications with providers during the process of clinical data exchange and feedback will be a critical component in the study of outcomes and application of the knowledge base. Efficient provider communications flow will be the energizing catalyst that elevates outcomes measurement to outcomes management, the process by which treatment practices will be continually measured, reviewed, tested, and redefined toward greater effectiveness, efficiency, and value. This broadened experience will influence all aspects of the daily operations of organized care delivery systems. Integrated communications and data management systems that supply a broad array of helpful care delivery components, such as patient eligibility data, clinical records, diagnostic assistance, claims payment, and educational updates, will upgrade quality management. Once providers are armed with accurate and detailed quality and treatment outcome data, there will be enormous progress in patient care. Behavioral health care administrators and the provider networks they manage will also benefit greatly. With more sophisticated quality measures, provider profiling and assessment functions will be improved, and the quality of the networks themselves will advance accordingly. An additional positive result that will accrue to the benefit of the health care system is that better quality care is often lower in cost due to efficiency, fewer complications, and better long-term results (Teisberg et al. 1994).

The transition to and establishment of outcomes management as a core quality improvement method will create opportunity for the psychiatric community.

When physicians work cooperatively in the design and implementation of quality and outcomes programs, they are much more likely to support such programs. And it is in an atmosphere of administrative cooperation and support that the knowledge level of the psychiatric profession will advance.

Public Mental Health Programs

With the likelihood that health care reform will expand both the behavioral coverages of and populations served by public programs that are already experiencing financial difficulties, managed behavioral health care will become increasingly important in that sector. Moreover, it is expected that national quality standards will cause the same demands for improved quality and accountability for care that exist in the private sector to occur in the public sector.

The more varied psychosocial needs and higher percentages of youth and the seriously and persistently mentally ill in public patient populations will require heavier involvement of the therapeutic and medication management skills of psychiatrists. From an administrative perspective, there will be considerable challenges in coordinating the expertise and capabilities of managed behavioral systems and existing public providers and facilities, such as state and VA hospitals and community mental health centers, in efficiently delivering care. The significant public-private differences in terms of funding sources and treatment settings and the need to reconcile the established systemic emphases of the two systems will punctuate the value of those having familiarity with and psychiatric experience in both sectors.

Furthermore, new opportunities in outcome research will arise as a greater potential to examine the effectiveness and efficiency of a broader range of treatment modalities and settings on outcomes is realized (Geraty and Fox 1996). Again, integrated behavioral systems will be the delivery vehicles that will have the human and technical resources required to manage the development, implementation, and evaluation of standardized protocols, guidelines, and other decision support mechanisms to improve the delivery of care.

Preparing for the Changing Delivery System

Proper preparation of the psychiatric profession for the realities of new delivery systems is a vital task in ensuring a well-functioning behavioral health care environment. There is a need to expose residents to administrative mechanisms and economic concerns early on in their training. Although some progress has been made, there is much room for improvement. It is anticipated that as a higher degree of cooperation and coordination between integrated delivery systems and academia develop as a part of outcomes research programs, the opportunities and advantages of more thorough training in managed care techniques will become much more evident. Such training will eliminate resistance to the unfamiliar and will increase the level of immediate contribution to the health care system.

For current members of the profession, a self-assessment of skills may be warranted. Most psychiatrists are not particularly fluent in the methods of developing policies and procedures, supervising quality improvement programs, and managing licensure and accreditation processes. Nor are psychiatrists generally well prepared to manage financial issues of the delivery system. As we move toward more sophisticated managed care systems for mental health and substance abuse care delivery, the need for more comprehensive administrative skills becomes even clearer. Six key areas where provider skills generally need improvement have been identified (Oss 1993):

- Management information systems
- Delivery system affiliation
- Utilization management
- Financial management
- Marketing
- Organizational leadership and staffing

In particular, the increasing complexities of quality and outcome data management call for further professional education in computer and communication systems skills. The managed behavioral health care industry has recognized the fundamental importance of provider education in this and other areas and is eager to work cooperatively with all appropriate educational institutions in further preparing the psychiatric profession for the challenges of tomorrow.

Back to the Future

As managed care organizations become more heavily integrated with providers, managers will become focused on the demonstration of value. By decreasing costs through the proper use of the entire continuum of care and through outcomes measurement and management, value will be significantly enhanced. Administrative psychiatrists, therefore, will be concentrating their greatest energies on a basic professional aspiration—expanding the discipline's store of knowledge in order to improve the quality of patient care. In that sense, developments in managed behavioral health care represent a return to the core of professional purpose. A clearer view of the changing health care system informs us that we need not turn our backs to the promise of evolving behavioral delivery methods but that we would do well to stride with renewed commitment toward the possibilities before us.

References

Bengen-Seltzer B: Industry analysis: delivery system trends affect behavioral health providers and MCOs. Open Minds 8(2):4–5, 1994a

Bengen-Seltzer B: Industry analysis: overlapping of managed care and provider roles in managed behavioral health evolution. Open Minds 8(4):4–5, 1994b

Berenson RA: A physician's view of managed care. Health Aff Winter: 106–119, 1991

Berenson RA: Do physicians recognize their own best interests? Health Aff Spring:185–193, 1994

Caton CL, Gralnick A: A review of issues surrounding length of psychiatric hospitalization. Hosp Community Psychiatry 38:858–863, 1987

Chandler D, Meisel J, McGowan M, et al: Client outcomes in two model capitated integrated service agencies. Psychiatr Serv 47:175–180, 1996

Crits-Cristoph P: The efficacy of brief dynamic psychotherapy: a meta-analysis. Am J Psychiatry 149:151–158, 1992

Dorwart RA, Chartock LR, Dial T, et al: A national study pf psychiatrist's professional activities. Am J Psychiatry 149:1499–1505, 1992

Etheredge L, Jones S: Managing a pluralist health system. Health Aff Winter:93–105, 1991

Geraty RD: The Impact of Managed Behavioral Healthcare on the Costs of Psychiatric and Chemical Dependency Treatment. Alexandria, VA, American Managed Behavioral Healthcare Association, 1994

Geraty RD, Fox RJ: Can managed care improve mental health outcomes for children and adolescents? in Controversies in Managed Mental Health Care. Edited by Lazarus A. Washington, DC, American Psychiatric Press, 1996

Gottlieb GL: Diversity, uncertainty, and variations in practice: the behaviors and clinical decisionmaking of mental health care providers, in The Future of Mental Health Services Research. Washington, DC, U.S. Department of Health and Human Services, 1989
Kane RA: Case management: ethical pitfalls on the road to high-quality managed care. Quality Review Bulletin 14:161–166, 1988
Marques C, Geraty R, Bartlett J, et al: Quality and access in the managed behavioral healthcare industry. Alexandria, VA, American Managed Behavioral Healthcare Association, 1994
Menninger RW: Administration and policy in mental health. Administration and Policy in Mental Health 21:107–112, 1993
Mental Health Weekly: In the search for effective measures, a quest for consensus. 4(28):2, 1994
Oss M: Industry analysis: how can behavioral health providers thrive in the managed care era? Open Minds 7, 1994
Physician Characteristics and Distribution in the U.S., 1994
Povar G: Hippocrates and the health maintenance organization. Ann Intern Med September 1988, pp. 419–424
Renz EA, Chung R, Fillman TO, et al: The effect of managed care on the treatment outcome of substance use disorders. Gen Hosp Psychiatry 17:287–292, 1995
Sperry L, Brill PL, Howard K, et al: Treatment Outcomes in Psychotherapy and Psychiatric Interventions. New York, Brunner-Mazel, 1996
Teisberg EO, Porter ME, Brown GB: Making competition in health care work. Harvard Business Review July–August, 1994
White J: Markets, budgets, and health care cost control. Health Aff Fall: 44–57, 1993

CHAPTER SIX

The Future of Private Office Practice of Psychiatry in an Environment Dominated by Managed Care

Norman A. Clemens, M.D.

Revolutionary changes in health care delivery are under way. Systems designers predict the demise of private psychiatric practice, viewed disdainfully as a cottage industry. Among many private psychiatrists a different view holds sway, intensified by what happens with their patients. They sense that eventually, beyond the current tumult, the demands of a discerning public will prevail and private psychiatric practice will survive.

As this chapter was written, there was great uncertainty about the direction that legislated health systems reform will take. Sweeping initiatives collapsed during the 1994 Congressional session. Subsequent Republican Congresses favored a minimal, incremental approach to insurance reform while privatizing Medicare and devolving Medicaid to the states. Some states are attempting health systems reform but encountering difficulties. A single-payer referendum failed in the 1994 California election by a large margin.

At the same time, the private health care system is in a tumultuous, headlong rush to managed care and organized systems. Private practitioners are feeling the pinch of selective contracting, pressures to form capitated bargaining units, and intrusive micromanagement of treatment decisions. Older psychiatrists have begun to count the years before retirement, whereas younger ones hesitate to embark on what they view as the risky enterprise of private practice. How can there be grounds for hope?

The Strengths of Private Practice

The answer rests on the intrinsic worth of private psychiatric practice. To begin with, it is *private*. Records and personal confidences remain with the psychiatrist, not a hospital record room or a central health care corporation computer system. Many private psychiatrists have no employees at all, whereas others hire someone part-time to help with appointments, correspondence, or billing. Besides the protection of privacy, this simplicity leads to a second great advantage, an economic one—the overhead costs of psychiatric private practice are minimal compared to most fields of medicine.

However, the most important advantage is the patient's direct, one-to-one, professionally grounded relationship with his or her psychiatrist. This dyadic foundation for effective treatment cannot be replaced by a team, an organization, or a triadic partnership with a managed care reviewer. It is hard to imagine a field of medicine where the physician's personal rapport, detailed knowledge over time, intensive therapeutic involvement, and continuity of work with the patient are more important in moments of crisis—often with highly cost-effective results in avoiding hospitalization or emergency-room expenses (Hoke 1989; Linehan et al. 1991, 1993). Furthermore, the governing values of treatment are directly accessible to the patient's ability to sense and explore them; they do not rest in the remote headquarters of a business organization. Such direct, personal, intuitive knowledge of the psychiatrist by the patient cannot be replaced by a statistical print-out or a "quality report card" when it comes to selecting a provider.

The psychiatrist-patient relationship is the vehicle for effective treatment. This is most obvious in psychoanalytic psychotherapy, in which long-standing difficulties come to light through repetition in the relationship with the therapist. Yet the individual relationship between doctor and patient may be equally important—sometimes to the point of being life-saving—in the case of chronic, serious illness such as schizophrenia, major affective disorders, or disabling personality disorders, where the predominant therapy may be medications and supportive management. Here the patient's ability to seek treatment in the face of overwhelming distortion of inner reality may rest on access to a trusted psychiatrist who has brought the patient through previous episodes.

Insight-oriented psychotherapies aim to help the patient eventually to resolve the transference and become independent of treatment. Yet the importance of this unique relationship is such that it is never forgotten. Follow-up studies in which psychoanalysts other than the treating analyst interviewed patients years after their treatment ended showed that the earlier transference awoke itself from dormancy with the new interviewer (Bachrach et al. 1991). Two thirds of "successfully analyzed" patients in one study contacted their analysts for brief interactions within three years of termination (Hartlaub et al. 1986). Child psychiatrists are accustomed to seeing their former patients for brief episodes during adolescence, as memories of childhood conflicts and transference phenomena surface and are re-mastered. Senior psychiatrists are accustomed to the return of patients decades after completion of psychotherapy at times of special stress such as the death of a parent, major narcissistic injury, or terminal illness. Some returning patients report referring routinely to their experience of psychotherapy in their coping with life during the long interval. With such patients, much can often be accomplished in a limited time.

In the current pressure toward organized systems, psychiatrists who work predominantly with outpatients are in an unique position compared to most other physicians because they generally do not require hospital and expensive technical services. The cost of outpatient psychiatric services is modest enough that many patients can choose to pay out of pocket rather than to involve themselves with their HMOs (Simon et al. 1994). Thus, outpatient psychiatrists have more options than other doctors as health systems changes unfold.

Private Practice Is Not Homogeneous

Private practice is commonly thought of in terms of solo, autonomous, self-employed, fee-for-service medicine. Yet some private psychiatrists practice in groups. Fifty percent of all psychiatrists participate in managed care (American Medical Association 1994), as do 36.5% of psychoanalysts, a group strongly oriented to private practice

(Brauer et al. 1993); younger psychiatrists participate more frequently. Even more accept utilization review by an indemnity insurer. Many private psychiatrists provide services as independent contractors to public or private agencies or other organized delivery systems, and some work as salaried employees of other private practitioners. Thus private psychiatrists have already shown their flexibility and resilience in adapting to changing health care delivery and financing systems, without losing the essential character of private practice. By definition one can say that the most common distinguishing feature of private practice is that the practitioner is primarily self-employed and autonomous.

Although many private practitioners utilize some form of psychotherapy as a major element of treatment of most patients, private practice is not synonymous with psychotherapy-oriented practice. A significant segment of private practitioners treats a patient population for whom medications, a supportive relationship, and psychiatric management rather than intensive psychotherapy are most likely to be the modal treatment plan, and for whom hospitalization is sometimes required. Nonetheless, defending access to effective psychotherapy has become an overriding concern to private practitioners as organized systems degrade the status of psychotherapy done by psychiatrists.

Systems Versus the Individual

The zeal for cost containment in the face of rising medical costs, coupled with intolerable inequities in health insurance coverage, has provoked an outcry for major changes in the health care system. Since experts in health care policy and administration, insurance, managed care, or management systems propose most of the remedies, it is not surprising that they value the imposition of organizational management and disparage the privately exercised judgment of individual doctors and patients. The result is great tension between the organizers and planners on the one hand and, on the other, the doctors and patients who live in clinical reality and cherish the sanctity of the private compact between them. Essentially, the new systems superimpose management controls that override trust in individual judgment based on professional ethics, ideals, and standards of practice that practitioners hold as a central core of their professional identity.

The causes of health-care cost inflation are often attributed to such broad trends as the medical successes that allow aging of a larger proportion of the population (Gaylin 1993), costly technological advances, cost-shifting from underfunded public programs and indigent care, high expectations and low cost-sharing by patients, malpractice litigation, and entrepreneurial abuses. Others take a "systemic view" that blames "incentives for private decision-makers to expand and intensify medical services," such as "overspecialization, overbuilding, and overspending" (Starr 1992).

Except for substance abuse treatment, the trend of inflation for treatment of mental illness has not been remarkable compared to health care costs in general (Hay/Huggins Co. 1991; Oss 1992). Nonetheless, a major element of managed care has aggressively and profitably tackled mental illness along with substance abuse, resulting in mental health managed care "carve-outs" that boast of reducing the portion of the health care dollar spent on these illnesses from a prevailing 8% (Hay/Huggins Co. 1991) level to as low as 3%–4% (Krizay 1990, Patterson 1992). This constitutes a new form of stigmatization and discrimination against the mentally ill.

Private practitioners sense a profound violation of conditions deemed essential to effective psychiatric treatment, especially treatment of entrenched, serious illness. These conditions are privacy and confidentiality, the fullest possible participation of the patient in treatment decisions, and the patient's confidence that the psychiatrist will act ethically in the patient's best interests and remain available as long as needed. Privacy must be maintained, even when confidentiality has been waived for insurance claim purposes, so that the patient can feel safe in divulging sensitive personal information without fear that it will cause damage in reputation, work, or relationships. Taking part in treatment decisions in the context of informed consent is a crucial initial step the patient makes toward taking charge of his or her illness and life patterns. Continuity is fundamental so that the strength of the relationship, not to speak of the wealth of data and experience the patient and the psychiatrist have accumulated together, will not be lost to the patient. Patients cannot be confident in exploring very sensitive and painful issues unless they are safe in the knowledge that their psychiatrists will see them through to resolution of what has been opened up. This principle has been recognized by the United States Supreme Court in *Jaffee v. Redmond* (Jaffee v Redmond 1996).

By their actions, systems managers subordinate these vital ingredients of effective treatment to financial and systemic considerations. Only rarely do psychiatrist-managers convey substantive concern about preserving the essential conditions for effective psychotherapy, as did Goldman when he spoke out for "continuity of therapist" and against the therapist-medicator split (Goldman 1994a).

Whereas the managers view the practitioners as intransigently resistant to change and accountability, the practitioners view the managers as posing a deadly threat to the fundamentals of their life work. The current state of high anxiety, sense of helplessness, depression, and rage among private practitioners is an understandable consequence. They feel that their integrity—in all the senses of the word—is threatened. One cannot overstate the intensity of their anger and frustrated desire to fight back.

The Apocalypse Has Begun . . .

In a market-driven frenzy, the organized systems are already sweeping across the country with explosive results in city after city. Enrollment in health maintenance organizations (HMOs) and preferred provider organizations (PPOs) grew to 149 million in 1995 (American Medical News 1996). Managed care has evolved from retrospective review to concurrent and prospective management (ranging from intrusive to coercive), and from discounted fee-for-service to capitation contracts. Hospitals and doctors are now forming vertically integrated multispecialty systems that assume insurance risk in order to regain local control of financial resources and patient care; primary care gatekeepers then control access to psychiatric services.

Production goals are being set: One university-related managed care system known to the author has proposed office and patient care standards to its professionals, requiring psychiatrists to see 2.25 patients per hour, while allowing psychologists the relatively indolent

The Future of Private Office Practice of Psychiatry   93

pace of 1.75 patients per hour! Gone there is the 45- to 50-minute hour; even the 30-minute session is in jeopardy. Managed care systems promulgate to their psychiatrists instructional materials comparing "progressive" with "regressive" techniques and principles in psychotherapy (Table 6–1). The preferred approach (based on an undocumented claim to "research evidence") clearly is designed to

Table 6–1. Working with a managed care company

Working with a managed care company such as HAI entails understanding the philosophy behind the treatment methods it supports, which can be placed on a continuum. The best available research evidence appears to support the superior efficacy of treatments characterized in this table as "progressive."

	Regressive ⟶	Progressive
Goals	• Vague and ambitious • Described as personality change or growth	• Specific and measurable • Focus on resolution
Assumptions of how change occurs	• Therapeutic relationship • Expressions of emotion	• Positive action on part of patient
Assumptions of dose/benefit	• More is better • Brief treatment as "Band-Aid"	• Creates gains in early sessions • Intermittent treatment as effective as continuous treatment
Expectations of patients	• Emotional relationship with therapist • Commitment to long duration of therapy	• Working relationship based on mutual trust • Commitment to work outside of treatment to reduce frequency and duration of treatment
Therapist behaviors	• Express emotional support • Interpretation	• Express confidence in patient's abilities • Teach and coach new skills/behavior

Source. Adapted from *Network Connection,* Human Affairs Intl/Aetna, November/December 1993.

discourage the kind of doctor-patient relationship in which trust, reliance on continuity and professional commitment, therapeutic engagement, transference, self-discovery, and modification of underlying psychopathology could emerge. Favored are directive and educational interventions that minimize free expression by the patient. The value-laden terms "progressive" and "regressive" preclude a balanced view of a range of valid techniques to be individualized to the needs of each patient; they disparage what some patients will inevitably require—intensive, exploratory work based on a secure relationship.

Some systems reportedly refuse to contract with or retain psychiatrists whose training and practice include long-term, insight-oriented psychotherapy. In pursuit of lower costs, organized systems are channeling patients to less-trained providers whose fees or salaries are lower (Jellinek 1993; Open Minds 1992; Weiner 1994).

In such systems, the psychiatrist's role is being narrowed to evaluation, medication management, hospital care, emergencies, and the outpatient treatment of patients who become severely ill despite lower-intensity ministrations—and away from psychotherapy (Thomas 1994). This is a familiar picture to almost anyone in private practice, certainly in urban areas. Staff model managed care organizations use about 4.3 psychiatrists per 100,000 population, in contrast to the 12.0 in the general U.S. supply in 1992 (Kronick 1993; Weiner 1994). In a capitated era one dire prediction is that 9,451 psychiatrists would be needed in the United States, in contrast to 36,405 practicing psychiatrists in 1993, a surplus of 26,954 or 74.0% (Advisory Board Co. 1993). In contrast, need-based GMENAC data project the need for about 55,000 psychiatrists in 2010 (Abt Associates Inc., undated). In some managed care systems a large proportion of psychiatrists has been abruptly dropped from managed care panels, with no evident regard for the resultant disruption of treatment relationships (OHIOMedicine 1994; Psychiatric News 1992). The remaining psychiatrists may be viewed as "trusted providers" who can be counted on to do limited treatment without micromanagement, or they may be given such volume that they have no time to conduct substantive psychotherapy.

The idealistic vision of managed care is to give whatever care is appropriate and necessary in the most cost-effective manner (Goldman

1994a, 1994b); this includes intensive and long-term care when deemed necessary (Paris 1994). Some managed care systems do aspire to accomplish this goal. However, most managed care firms appear to have entered into intense price competition based on draconian cost cutting. Yet, premium dollars are diverted from services to patients into administrative overhead of 12.3% (American Medical News 1994), shareholder earnings such as 6.6%–9.4% (Open Minds 1992, 1994), high executive salaries (Washington Post 1994), and massive corporate equity: In 1993 Value Health bought out Preferred HealthCare for $425,000,000. An independent audit of Ohio Biodyne operations showed that only $4.7 million out of $14 million premiums in 1991–1992 was spent on patient care (Wall Street Journal 1995). The value of mergers and acquisitions involving health care companies in 1994 rose to $19.9 billion (Securities Data Company 1994). Advertising expenditures by health and dental insurers in the first nine months of 1994 were $180 million, up from $106 million in the same period the year before (Competitive Media Reporting 1994). The financial and legal power of the huge insurance companies that are predicted to dominate the health care scene, coupled with anti-trust restraints on self-employed physicians, leave the individual private practitioner totally overmatched.

Financial incentives other than managed care also push the private practitioner toward spending a much smaller proportion of practice time in 45- to 50-minute sessions of psychotherapy. Reimbursement schedules, particularly those based on the Harvard Resource-Based Relative Value Scale and its deviant offspring, the Medicare Fee Schedule, strongly favor payment for the codes for medication management and even brief psychotherapy over reimbursement for individual medical psychotherapy, 45–50 minutes, or medical psychoanalysis. The private practitioner can clearly make more money doing medication management and giving electroconvulsive treatments (Lewin-VHI, Inc. 1993). There is already striking evidence that patterns of practice are changing correspondingly (Mucha 1994).

Changes in the work force further reduce the likelihood that many young psychiatrists will set up solo private practices. Since 1988 the number of U.S. medical school graduates entering psychiatric training through the National Residents Matching Program has fallen by 41% (Scully 1994). Various reasons have been proposed to explain this decline, ranging from the low income of psychiatrists to deemphasis of patient care in the more academically prestigious, research-oriented medical schools.

Other environmental shifts favor the entrance of young psychiatrists into organized systems rather than private practice. Huge medical school debts may prevent students from borrowing the capital needed to set up an office. The need for hospital affiliations in order to become known and build up a practice will be a powerful pressure toward becoming an employee rather than a private practitioner, as the hospitals race to form and control integrated hospital-physician organizations. As the proportion of women in medical school classes approaches 50%, and as new physicians in general place more of a premium on family life, there may be a greater trend to choose employment over independent practice because of the advantages of structured working hours and flexibility for child care.

All of these changes point toward a diminution of the amount of psychiatric service that takes place in solo private practice settings. Other trends are more favorable.

... But There Are Opportunities

Team approaches to the case management of certain conditions (such as severe and persistent mental illness) and populations (such as children and adolescents) offer opportunities for enterprising private practitioners. These are enhanced by the growing trend toward privatization of the care of the severely ill in what is often spoken of as a "public-private partnership." These situations will call on the psychiatrist to employ or form collaborative relationships with professionals from other disciplines to provide medical, social, legal, financial, and vocational services in an integrated environment on a contract basis with public mental health agencies. The model closely resembles the psychiatrically grounded community mental health model (Joint Commission on Mental Illness and Health 1961). Combining the best of the private doctor-patient relationship and coordinated multidisciplinary services may raise the care of the severely and persistently mentally ill to a new level. Child and adolescent psychiatrists have a long history of providing coordinated, multidisciplinary care for their patients and their parents, and so contracting with an integrated system may not require unduly difficult adjustments for a collaborative practice group.

Opposing Trends

Some of the failed national health systems reform bills would have provided some solace for beleaguered private practitioners. During the great health systems debate of 1994, Congress was heavily bombarded with objections to managed care. Mandated availability of fee-for-service and point-of-service options would have allowed patients to choose private offices over organized settings. Regulations might have curbed the more damaging forms of managed care intrusion on the doctor-patient relationship. Systems that established competition within standardized, defined parameters of quality treatment could have shifted the balance toward forcing organized systems to compete on the basis of genuine quality rather than overly aggressive cost containment. Genuine quality would have to include allowance for long-term treatment of serious illness.

Under the "managed competition" of the Clinton plan, organized systems would not have been so easily able to skim off the healthier patients, leaving those more in need of expensive services to burden the beleaguered indemnity plans. Because they would probably have had to care for a population of subscribers over an extended period, they would have found it to their advantage to provide intensive mental health services that require expenditures in the initial years but offer genuine savings in medical cost-offset in future years (Holder and Blose 1985, 1987; McDonnell Douglas Corporation 1989; Wall Street Journal 1989).

Market forces have subsequently brought about a significant increase in plans offering point-of-service options that allow subscribers to obtain services from professionals outside the roster of a managed care company, usually with an additional copayment. The public reactions to managed care have prompted the introduction of state and federal legislation to regulate managed care and protect consumers. These developments are favorable to private psychiatric practice.

A limited trial of medical savings accounts (MSAs) is taking place as a result of the health care reform legislation of 1996. These tax-deferred moneys are meant to be spent on services falling under a high deductible threshold before health insurance takes effect. Though paying for first-dollar care is expected to be an incentive to the consumer to spend less on medical care, it is likely that patients who value private, undisturbed psychiatric treatment will seek it out, making MSAs a boon to private psychiatric practice.

Outcomes Data Favor Private Practice

As organized systems shift psychotherapy to the least trained providers and hence away from psychiatrists, the results of this may work adversely to the patients of those systems. Psychiatrists have the unique advantage of being licensed physicians who do comprehensive evaluations. Their whole training has prepared them to understand the interaction of psyche and soma and the subjective experience of living within a body. They have special expertise with medication as well as psychotherapy. They share in a deeply held tradition that goes back to the ancient Greeks governing ethics, dedication to learning, and responsibility to patients. Patients place great trust and high expectations in this tradition. Clinical experience suggests that some patients within managed systems resent receiving only medication management from psychiatrists and being shunted to nonmedical professionals for psychotherapy, or getting only directive, formula-based psychotherapy that does not permit them to explore freely what they think and feel. So, on their own, they seek out a psychiatric physician who will talk with them. A survey is needed to corroborate or refute this clinical impression.

Evidence is now emerging that fee-for-service practice results in better patient outcomes. An incidental finding of the McDonnell Douglas study was that private practice patients had far better results in maintaining job stability than those referred to HMOs (McDonnell Douglas Corporation 1989). In a Rand Corporation study depressed patients treated by private psychiatrists showed symptomatic and functional improvement, whereas HMO patients worsened or remained on a plateau (Rogers et al. 1993). The traditional expression of outcomes assessment, which will probably never be supplanted by management "report cards," is word-of-mouth among satisfied patients. If affordable fee-for-service, point-of-service and medical-savings-account alternatives to managed care remain in the system, the marketplace of the real "consumers"—the patients and their families—may well favor the private practitioner. One study of HMO patients showed that 5% used mental health services within the HMO and 9% used services outside the HMO system (Simon et al. 1994).

The Public Backlash Intensifies

As employers and Medicaid programs force more and more people into managed care, a public backlash is emerging. News magazines warn against HMO abuses and interference with trust in the doctor-patient relationship (Newsweek 1995; Time 1996), including HMO obstructions to access to psychotherapy (Spragins 1997). Independent consumer studies show that many HMOs fall short of their promises (Consumer Reports 1996) and that consumers experience longer-term psychotherapy (usually shunned by managed care) as being more beneficial than short-term treatment (Consumer Reports 1995). Reports of high HMO profits, massive executive compensation (New Haven Register 1996), rising administrative costs (Woolhandler et al. 1991), lack of choice of physician or hospital, difficulties in obtaining treatment of serious or unusual diseases (Rosenthal 1996), and incentives to physicians to withhold treatment (Pear 1996)—all enhance public distrust and resistance to managed care.

But the public outrage is greatest against egregious violations of the doctor-patient relationship, such as "gag clauses" in managed care contracts that forbid doctors to discuss freely with patients the full range of treatment options, covered or not, or to reveal financial incentives or difficulties connected with the plan itself (Herbert 1996). Trust in doctors is eroding (Kaveny et al. 1996). The public outcry has resulted not only in competitive pressure to correct abuses but also in legislation in many states to regulate managed care entities (Jenkins 1996; Kuttner 1996). In late 1996 a presidential Advisory Commission on Consumer Protection and Quality in the Health Care Industry proposed a medical Consumer Bill of Rights and Responsibilities (available at http://www.whitehouse.gov), which President Clinton promptly applied to federal health plans and challenged Congress to enact into law. If such trends result in protection of the doctor-patient relationship and the Hippocratic tradition, private psychiatrists may be able to work more comfortably in contractual arrangements with organized systems.

Entering the New Marketplace

The privacy, autonomy, simplicity, flexibility, and direct relationships with patients that private practice affords will always appeal to many psychiatrists, as long as it is legally permissible for them to practice independently. Psychiatrists will choose this path even if financial sacrifices are necessary to broaden the potential referral base of patients.

Will the 45- to 50-minute hour survive? Dedication to psychoanalytic therapies and the satisfaction derived from their beneficial effects on patients will sustain a cadre of psychiatrists who will be sought out for their expertise. Even in Czechoslovakia under Communist domination, the teaching and practice of psychoanalysis persisted as an underground activity (Beigler 1994).

Private hospital practice for patients with severe illness who want privacy and autonomy will also have a powerful appeal, especially to those in highly visible occupations that are sensitive to public opinion. Privacy concerns in the current environment of high information transfer and low security cause many high executives and public figures to pay out of pocket for office treatment rather than risk embarrassment through disclosure of insurance claims.

Private practice of psychiatry can survive in several possible scenarios. Established psychiatrists in the later years of their career, with a largely self-paying clientele, may be able to continue much as they are, as may psychiatrists in sparsely populated areas. Psychiatrists early in their careers will have to make major accommodations and perhaps go through several stages. Some hypothetical scenarios follow.

1. *Employment early in a psychiatric career in order to pay off debts, with private practice at a later career stage.* This career path has traditionally been used by many psychiatrists who initially worked in full-time academic or hospital positions, the military, the Public Health Service, or state and community systems before entering private practice. If staff-model HMOs pursue a path of recruiting young psychiatrists by paying them well, this mode of entry into clinical practice will be very common. Whether employed psychiatrists will eventually migrate into autonomous private practice will be influenced by whether they find work within organized systems to be professionally satisfying.

2. *Employment part time, coexistent with part-time private practice.* This too is a relatively common mode used for generations by psychiatrists in various academic, administrative, and public system positions. Employment may range from a day or two a week, with the balance being private practice, to six or eight hours a day, allowing time for a few private patients in the early morning or evening. It remains to be seen to what extent organized systems will permit such division of practice time and venue.

3. *Independent contracting of private practitioners with IPAs and PPOs,* along with seeing self-paying and indemnity-insured patients in full-time office practice. This is becoming the current modal situation. In 1993 approximately half of all psychiatrists participated in managed care contracts (in contrast to 75% of all physicians) (American Medical Association 1993). If managed care enrollment grew rapidly along with constriction of psychiatrist panels in organized systems, a surplus of psychiatrists would be in intense competition for the remaining indemnity-insured and self-paying patients.

4. *Participation in vertically integrated, multispecialty hospital/ physician groups that are capitated for primary care but pay fees for independent specialty services.* This mode of practice is likely to be subject to primary care gatekeeper constrictions and

discounted fees. Its advantages are the integration of primary care and psychiatric services and the visibility of the resultant cost offsets through reduced medical costs for psychiatric patients. The quality of psychiatric services would depend heavily on the nature of the relationship of the specialist with the primary care provider, especially if the payment for specialty services is included as a cost-containment device in the gatekeeper's capitated insurance risk. Here the advantage of local control carries with it the continuing obligation to educate and negotiate with each primary care provider, whose fiscal incentives may foster delaying referral and inappropriately prescribing medication without the early advantage of proper clinical assessment, knowledge of psychopharmacology, and psychotherapy skills that the well-trained psychiatrist offers.

5. *Formation and control of mental health provider groups to contract and set terms of treatment as a mental health carve-out unit, most likely on a risk-sharing, capitated basis.* This option of joining in the evolution toward organized systems is predicted to occur on a large scale in the next few years. Its advantage is that contracted funding for mental health services might be protected from erosion by financial pressures in the rest of a managed medical system. Forming a capitated carve out may allow private practitioners to negotiate and preserve the environment for effective treatment, intensive when necessary. As IPAs they may be able to contract with employers who especially value the advantages private practitioners offer. However, forming more cohesively organized groups or entering into capitated contracts in price-competitive situations could place them under the same pressures that now exist in managed care and that compel them to fall back on short-term, directive, and less definitive approaches; to employ less-trained professionals; and to fragment the psychiatrist's relationship with patients by delegating psychotherapy to others. In this evolution toward corporate structures, the motivations, ethics, and standards of medical practice risk being eclipsed by those of private enterprise. The integrity of the private psychiatrist will be challenged in new ways.

6. *Totally independent fee-for-service practice on a self-paying basis, outside the third-party payment system.* Some psychiatrists see this as likely to be the only safe way, under most of the highly centralized reform schemes, to offer effective psychodynamic treatment; others disagree. This option assumes that the health care system will continue to permit private contracting or consider some services to be uncovered under the system and that patients and doctors will be free to make their own clinical and financial arrangements without government interference. The right to contract privately must include giving the patient the freedom to forego use of existing coverage for services because of unacceptable conditions attached to the coverage—a choice that current Medicare regulations strongly discourage. Except for some reduced fee or pro bono work, this practice option would essentially be part of a multitiered system in which ability to pay would largely govern access to services unavailable within the standard health scheme.

Credo or Accurate Perception of the Marketplace?

This chapter began with an expression of faith: that patients would seek out private psychiatrists and support the continuance of private psychiatric practice. Unless a highly coercive, organized system were to emerge from reform legislation and the freedom of doctors and patients to contract privately outside the system were to be abolished, it is difficult to conceive that there would not be self-paying patients seeing private psychiatrists.

The scenario for an individual's practice within the third-party payment system depends on many variables. The higher the degree of dependence any provider has on third-party payment—particularly for hospital work—and the higher the degree of penetration of capitated, organized systems, the more likely it is that many private psychiatrists will be forced to become employees or highly controlled independent contractors or even to leave the field. The emergence of a single-payer system, widely available medical savings accounts, or a strong, affordable, minimally managed fee-for-service/point-of-service option within managed systems would provide autonomous private practice a better opportunity for healthy longevity. If organized systems can find a way genuinely to integrate and preserve the strengths of private practice, such as true privacy, choice of therapist, participation of the patient in treatment decisions, and secure continuity of the treatment relationship, then patients and dedicated practitioners may find a congenial place in organized settings.

In any case, the human desire for freedom, privacy, and control over one's own life must inevitably be a force driving patients to seek the great advantages that the private psychiatrist offers. Patients with serious, recurrent illnesses who want the assurance of a steady, confidential, one-to-one relationship will seek out private psychiatrists. Psychiatrists known for being physicians with special expertise in intensive psychotherapy will continue to be sought out by discerning patients, even those with limited resources, who know that their best hope lies in that form of treatment, with or without medications. Private practice will survive and perhaps even thrive, albeit in a different manner from its previous dominant role in the treatment of mental illness.

References

Abt Associates Inc.: Physician characteristics and distribution in the U.S. Chicago, IL, American Medical Association (not dated)

Advisory Board Co.: Capitation I: The New American Medicine. Advisory Board Co. 1993

American Medical Association: Data graphed in Most doctors in managed care. USA Today, June 13, 1994, A8

American Medical News: HMOs boomed in '93. October 10, 1994, p 5

American Medical News: HMOs, PPOs cover 149 million Americans. July 22, 1996, p 2

Bachrach HM, Galatzer-Levy R, Skolnikoff A, Waldron S Jr: On the efficacy of psychoanalysis. J Am Psychoanal Assoc 39:871–916, 1991

Beigler, J: Personal communication on presentation of Professor Michael Subek, director of the Prague Psychoanalytic Institute, on "Psychoanalytic work with Jewish Holocaust survivors under the Communist regime" to the Chicago Psychoanalytic Institute, February 2, 1994

Brauer LD, Brauer S: Survey of psychoanalytic practice. American Psychoanalytic Association, 1993
Competitive Media Reporting, quoted in Erik Eckholm: While Congress remains silent, health care transforms itself. New York Times, December 18, 1994, pp 1, 34
Consumer Reports: Mental health: does therapy help? November 1995, pp 734–739
Consumer Reports: How good is your health plan? August 1996, pp 28–42
Gaylin W: Faulty diagnosis. Harper's Magazine, October 1993, pp 57–64
Goldman WH: Quoted in Managed care can improve services—or threaten them, says expert. Psychiatric News, August 19, 1994a, p 1
Goldman WH: In Managed care strategies discussed to aid private practitioners. APA Symposia Highlights on the Treatment of Depressive Disorders, SmithKline Beecham Pharmaceuticals, 1994b, pp 2, 10
Hartlaub GH, Martin GC, Rhine MW: Recontact with the analyst following termination: a survey of seventy-one cases. J Am Psychoanal Assoc 34: 895–910, 1986
Hay/Huggins Co., Inc.: Psychiatric health care benefits, studies conducted for the American Psychoanalytic Association and the National Association of Private Psychiatric Hospitals, 1991
Herbert B: Hidden agenda. New York Times, July 13, 1996, A13
Hoke LA: Longitudinal patterns of behaviors in borderline personality disorder. Unpublished doctoral dissertation. Boston University Graduate School, Boston, MA, 1989
Holder HD, Blose JO: Longitudinal analysis of health care utilization and costs for enrollees under the Aetna federal employees health benefits plan. National Institute of Alcoholism and Alcohol Abuse, 1985
Holder HD, Blose JO: Changes in health care costs and utilization associated with mental health treatment. Hosp Community Psychiatry 38:10, 1987
Jaffee v Redmond, (1996)
Jellinek MS, Nurcombe B: Two wrongs don't make a right: managed care, mental health, and the marketplace. JAMA 270:1737–1739, 1993
Jenkins HW Jr: Managed care suffers a bad case of politics. Wall Street Journal, July 16, 1996, A11
Joint Commission on Mental Illness and Health: Action for Mental Health: Final Report of the Joint Commission on Mental Illness and Health. Basic Books, New York, 1961
Kaveny MC, Lanagan JP: The doctor's call. New York Times, July 15, 1996, A11
Krizay J: Open Minds, April, 1990, p 8

Kronick R: The marketplace in healthcare reform: the demographic limitations of managed competition. N Engl J Med, January 14, 1993

Kuttner R: States fill the vacuum on health reform. Boston Globe, July 29, 1996, A15

Lewin-VHI, Inc., Annual incomes for psychiatrists under alternative practice scenarios and alternative payment scenarios. Report to American Psychiatric Association, 1993

Linehan MM, Armstrong HE, Suarez A: Cognitive-behavioral treatment of chronically parasuicidal borderline patients. Arch Gen Psychiatry 48:1060–1064, 1991

Linehan MM, Heard HL, Armstrong HE: Naturalistic follow-up of a behavioral treatment for chronically parasuicidal borderline patients. Arch Gen Psychiatry 50:971–974, 1993

McDonnell Douglas Corporation and Alexander & Alexander Consulting Group: Employee assistance program financial offset study, 1985–1988. 1989

Mucha T: Unpublished data on psychotherapy at Institute of Living, presentations at Western New England Psychoanalytic Society, March 26, 1994, and at American Academy of Psychoanalysis, May 21, 1994

New Haven Register: Aetna merger brings windfall to 7. June 14, 1996, D1

OHIOMedicine: Managed-care news around the state: Cincinnati . . . Psychiatrists dropped. July 1994, p 20

Open Minds: Industry statistics: psychiatrist share of outpatient behavioral health market drops to 22%. 1992

Open Minds: April 1992, p 8 (Re: Preferred Health Care); November 1992, p 1 (Re: Biodyne); April 1994, p 1 (Re: Value Health)

Oss M: Are behavioral health costs out of control? Open Minds, September 1992

Paris M, Ohio Medical Director, Medco Behavioral Care Systems Corp.: Presentation to Ohio Psychiatric Association, October 16, 1994

Patterson D: Quoted in Spending urged for HMO mental health care. American Medical News, February 3, 1992, p 8

Pear R: U.S. shelves plan to limit rewards to H.M.O. doctors; industry wins reprieve. New York Times, July 8, 1996, p 1

Psychiatric News: Psychiatrists allegedly locked out of Blue Cross plan. November 2, 1992, p 8

Rogers WH, Wells KB, Meredith LS, et al.: Outcomes for adult outpatients with depression under prepaid or fee-for-service financing. Arch Gen Psychiatry 50:517–525, 1993

Rosenthal E: Patients with rare illnesses fight new H.M.O.s to get treatment. New York Times, July 15, 1996, A1

Scully JH: Psychiatry workforce and health care reform. Washington, DC, Office of Education, American Psychiatric Association, 1994

Securities Data Company, reported in Erik Eckholm: While Congress remains silent, health care transforms itself. New York Times, December 18, 1994, pp 1, 34

Simon GE, VonKorff M, et al: Predictors of outpatient mental health utilization by primary care patients in a health maintenance organization. Am J Psychiatry 151:908–913, 1994

Spragins EE: Beware your HMO. Newsweek, October 23, 1995, p 54

Spragins EE: Shortchanging the psyche: will your HMO be there if you need therapy? Newsweek, August 25, 1997, p 78

Starr P: The logic of health-care reform: transforming American medicine for the better. Grand Rounds Press, Whittle Direct Books, 1992

Thomas S, Office of Economic Affairs, American Psychiatric Association: Unpublished data from the managed care hotline, 1994

Time: The soul of an HMO. January 22, 1996, pp 44–52

Wall Street Journal: Spending to cut mental-health costs (a report of the McDonnell Douglas study). December 13, 1989, B1

Wall Street Journal: Cost-cutting firms monitor couch time as therapists fret. July 13, 1995, A1, A3

Washington Post: Hill probe questions Blue Cross spending. August 5, 1994, B1

Weiner JP: Forecasting the effects of health reform on US physician workforce requirements: evidence from HMO staffing patterns. JAMA 272:222–230, 1994

Woolhandler S, Himmelstein DU: The deteriorating administrative efficiency of the U.S. health care system. N Engl J Med 324:1253–1258, 1991

Section III
Training, Guidelines, and Ethics

CHAPTER SEVEN

Psychiatric Training and Managed Care

James E. Sabin, M.D.

The Challenge

This chapter addresses the question of whether robust psychiatric training will be possible in an environment dominated by managed care.

To begin with the conclusion—I am certain that the answer is "yes," but only if psychiatric leaders can create a yet-to-be-established degree of collaboration between academic psychiatry and managed behavioral health care. To accomplish this, our profession will have to find new ways of integrating patient-centered and population-centered care and new ways of interacting with a health care system preoccupied with the bottom line.

Successful psychiatric training programs require four ingredients: science, patients, money, and a powerful vision of the future of the field.

Academic psychiatry has been the primary domain for development of psychiatry's scientific base since World War II. The biological, psychological, and social science bases of psychiatry are evolving rapidly, providing great potential benefit for our patients.

Managed behavioral health care systems have taken responsibility for the care of progressively larger groups of patients and control of the funds for that care since approximately 1980. By the end of the century, funding and service delivery will be controlled largely by managed care systems.

Without a powerful vision of what psychiatry can do and the roles psychiatrists will play in the future, the field will not attract talented trainees. This vision will emerge only if academic and managed care leaders can join together in coparenting it. Clearly, all those who care about robust psychiatric training programs and professionally satisfying roles for future psychiatrists need to encourage the academic psychiatry and managed behavioral health care sectors to collaborate.

Exhortation, however, will not do much to make this happen because academic psychiatry and managed behavioral health care already have strong reasons to cooperate. In addition to needing access to the patient populations and funds controlled by managed behavioral health care for its training programs, academic psychiatry needs markets for the graduates of those programs and its research findings. Managed behavioral health care cannot achieve its objective of enhancing what the British National Health Service calls "value for money" without the research on illness, treatment effectiveness, epidemiology, and health services conducted by academic psychiatry. In addition, although there is no shortage of psychiatrists at present, over time organized systems will require newly trained psychiatrists whose skills prepare them for high-quality, managed care practice.

As so often occurs in psychotherapy, the rate-limiting factor impeding progress is resistance, not desire. Facilitating the collaboration necessary for successful future training requires removal of barriers more than lighting of motivational fires.

Academic Psychiatry: Barriers to Collaboration With Managed Behavioral Health Care

Academic psychiatry and the American Psychiatric Association are currently losing power. Until recently, psychiatrists set the agenda for the mental health care system. Now those who pay for care—businesses and government—call the shots.

This transformation is part of a larger shift in the implicit contract between society and the professions. In medicine and psychiatry, we are increasingly being held accountable for meeting societal objectives, including cost containment. The current strategy in the United States for achieving these objectives is to encourage market forces in health care.

When payers decided to change the balance of power in mental health care, they created a new market. Managed behavioral health care responded to that market challenge. Academic and organized psychiatry—like Achilles in his tent at Troy—largely stayed on the sidelines. This decision has led to turmoil and massive demoralization in the profession.

Managed behavioral health care has been the agent of the enormous changes and the direct source of pain for the psychiatric profession. Because professions, like individuals, respond to change and narcissistic injury of this magnitude with anxiety, rage, and transient failures of reality testing, it is not surprising that academic and organized psychiatry initially both attacked and ignored managed behavioral health care in the hope that it would go away.

This reflexive attack-the-messenger response has been—and continues to be—the major barrier to potential collaboration between academic psychiatry and managed behavioral health care. The major antidotes are time and empathic leadership. Leaders need to help psychiatrists do what Elvin Semrad told residents to do with their patients: *Acknowledge* that change is truly happening and the pain associated with that change; provide help in *bearing* the pain; and put the process *into perspective* in order to move on constructively (Rako and Mazer 1980).

It may be wishful thinking on my part, but I believe that as of the summer of 1995 academic psychiatry appears to have turned a corner in its response to the new managed care environment. The largest current psychiatric residency—the Harvard Longwood Psychiatry Training Program—includes a health maintenance organization (HMO) (the Harvard Community Health Plan) as one of its five sponsors. The Department of Psychiatry at Duke University has launched a new journal that attempts to bridge the gap between the ivory tower and the new practice settings (Frances 1995). Finally, the American Association of Chairmen of Departments of Psychiatry and the American Association of Directors of Psychiatric Residency Training convened a three-day meeting with managed care leaders in August 1995 to consider new collaborative approaches to residency training.

The second barrier to collaboration has been a perceived incompatibility of values. Academic psychiatry commonly teaches that skillful and ethical psychiatrists should always make the optimal care of the individual patient their absolute value. In this spirit Dr. Jerome Kassirer, editor-in-chief of the *New England Journal of Medicine,* stated that "cost should never be a factor in the one-on-one encounter of a doctor and a patient" (Kassirer 1995).

If cost were truly the bottom line for all managed behavioral health care programs, academic psychiatry would be correct in refusing to work with managed care (Gabbard 1992). However, if I am correct in believing that ethical managed care systems seek to *maximize* outcomes (value) for an insured population, not simply to *minimize* expenditure on the individual patient, academic programs can be criticized for being slow to adopt a population-based ethics of stewardship to supplement the traditional Hippocratic fiduciary commitment to the individual patient (Sabin 1993).

Here too I believe there are signs of a more nuanced exploration of values that goes beyond polarized broadsides (by academic and organized psychiatry) against managed care per se as an ethical abomination and (by managed care) against academic psychiatry per se as ivory tower profligacy and elitism (Schreter, et al. 1994).

Managed Behavioral Health Care: Barriers to Collaboration With Academic Psychiatry

Practicing psychiatrists and academic programs often apply terms like "demanding," "arbitrary," and "controlling" to managed behavioral health care. Behind closed doors, however, managed behavioral health care leaders apply the same terms to the corporate and government purchasers who buy their "products." In the mid-1990s, clinicians, academics, managed behavioral health care-niks, and purchasers all regard the health care environment as threatening, difficult to influence, and "out of control."

Academic psychiatry smarts from loss of money and power. I believe the managed behavioral health care sector smarts from recurrently being characterized—by academic and organized psychiatry—as a rapacious, Judas-like betrayer who abandons patients and Hippocratic values for the sake of profit. These heated, often heartfelt, assaults create the first barrier to collaboration for training.

If managed behavioral health care did not need academic psychiatry, it might simply take its golden marbles and play elsewhere. But the need exists, so it cannot. Here, too, as with academic psychiatry, those who care about future psychiatric training must hope for visionary leaders who will not let the history of combative and condescending rhetoric about managed care prevent cooperative search for areas of mutual interest and potential collaboration.

I deliberately put money second on the list of barriers. The 1990s are clearly a decade of diminishing social investment of all kinds. Along with a host of other educational, environmental, and social welfare activities, medical education and psychiatric training will suffer. Borus provides the best analysis of economic influences on psychiatric education (Borus 1994). A national survey 10 years from now will almost certainly show an overall decline in the size and number of psychiatric training programs.

Managed behavioral health care is the means purchasers have chosen to constrain their expenditures and enhance the effectiveness of the money they spend. Its mandate is to manage mental health expenditures, not to oppose education and training. If purchasers asked the managed behavioral health care sector to support and promote education, it would do so with the same alacrity it shows in creating new clinical networks.

In other words, although the decreased funding associated with managed care is the most severe practical barrier to future psychiatric training, ensuring robust training in the future could quite properly be reframed as a problem *for* academic psychiatry and managed behavioral health care to solve rather than as a problem *between* them. Even if this collaborative reframing of the relationship between the academic and managed care sectors does not produce substantial new funding, it could facilitate other positive training developments. The next section suggests what some of these might be.

Four Objectives for Collaboration

1. *Make academic programs more cost competitive.* Academically based clinical programs can rarely compete on the basis of price with com-

munity programs that do not carry the cost of trainees, teaching time, and the higher severity of illness typically seen at academic sites. Although academic programs have lowered costs by reducing length of stay, improving productivity through efficiencies and increased work expectations, and downsizing, community programs have taken similar steps and retain a price advantage.

Following the example of industries in which producers join with their suppliers to improve the production process, managed behavioral health care firms ("producers") and academically based clinical programs ("suppliers") could join in trying to make the academic program a more viable preferred provider. If academic programs become part of larger networks, they could be used for the highly complex patients and clinical problems for which their expertise is a distinct value. Within the network, residents could have components of their training at community sites, ensuring a properly broad base of clinical experience during training. At present, managed behavioral health care firms allow academically based service programs to submit bids for participation in the network. In the collaborative framework I envision, the two sectors would work together to create a proposal that could meet both of their interests.

2. *Make services delivered by residents reimbursable.* To date, many managed behavioral health care networks have refused to pay for services delivered by psychiatric residents. Collaborative problem solving can take us a long way with this difficult issue.

Corporate and government purchasers of health insurance are rarely interested in micromanaging the ways in which services are delivered. Their appropriate concerns are with the quality and cost of the services provided to the insured population and the population's satisfaction with the care it receives. In meetings with the managed care committee of the American Psychiatric Association, the medical directors of several of the largest managed behavioral health care companies have stated that if they were confident that an academic program in which psychiatric residents delivered services could give proper assurance regarding quality of care, purchasers would accept the training program as part of the service network.

Simple assurances, however, will not provide the necessary confidence. In the past, training programs have given residents extraordinary latitude to conduct treatment independently. Although this degree of autonomy may enhance professional identity and certainly allows experiential learning, it is not compatible with responsible managed behavioral health care.

In designing service programs in which residents provide care, academic leaders should ask themselves two questions. First, to address the issue of quality—"what design features would make me comfortable with members of my own family receiving their treatment in this program?" Having posed this question to many training directors, I can report that the answer virtually always involves stipulations about the degree of responsibility the attending or supervising psychiatrist would have to take. The second question clarifies how that responsibility should be exercised: "If I took residents into my own personal practice, and my livelihood depended on the quality and professional reputation of that practice, how would I work with the residents?"

In 1994–1995 I was able to apply these design principles to two six-month placements of half-time PGY III residents in my own outpatient practice in the staff model division of the Harvard Community Health Plan HMO. In order to meet my commitment to the clinical chief and to my own sense of responsibility (the patients the residents treated were defined by the HMO as part of *my* practice), I wanted the residents to observe me so they could see how I felt patients should be treated, and I wanted to observe them to make sure this was happening. Whereas in typical individual supervision I would follow a subgroup of a resident's patients through discussion during the supervisory hour, in the HMO placement I needed to know about every patient and be available for consultation outside of the regularly scheduled supervisory time. I felt responsible not just for ensuring that the treatment was safe and technically correct but also that the patients felt well cared for (in the jargon of managed care, this is called "member satisfaction") and that the rest of the team found the residents to be positive colleagues.

This is the kind of supervision and quality assurance that would allow a managed behavioral health care company to reimburse for services delivered by residents. The overall situation embodies what educators will recognize as a familiar form of parallel process. If the academic site can assure the managed care program regarding the quality of care delivered to the patients treated by residents, the managed care program will be able to provide comparable assurance to its purchasers about the quality of care that will be delivered to the insured population. To a substantial degree, the problem of making services delivered by residents reimbursable should be improved by careful collaborative planning.

3. *Make academic programs high-value service sites.* As purchasers become more experienced and as managed behavioral health care systems mature, purchasing transactions will focus more on "value" (quality plus cost) than cost alone. This movement from cost-based to value-based purchasing opens a competitive possibility for academic programs. Academically based clinical programs may cost more than community alternatives, but if their quality is demonstrably higher, they may be seen as providing greater overall value.

In the past, society generally took the medical profession's word regarding the definition of high-quality care. That trust continues in large degree in individual patient-doctor interactions. Purchasers and the managed care enterprises that serve them are well aware of the studies of practice variation, however, and regularly insist that quality must be demonstrated.

Unfortunately, it is extraordinarily difficult to demonstrate quality in a rigorous manner. The problem has two components: 1) defining the dimensions of quality in ways that can be measured and 2) doing the measurement.

Academically based service programs, as "suppliers" of clinical care, need to know what the managed care "customer" wants to buy. In circumstances of collaboration, the managed care and academic partners will work together to define the important dimensions of quality. In these discussions the academic partner will (and should) advocate for professionally based standards of excellence, and the managed care partner will (and should) advocate for identifying and satisfying the concerns of the purchaser.

The old joke—"the operation was a success, but, unfortunately, the patient died"—warns us of the danger of overemphasizing technical definitions of quality. The more recent joke—"the cheapest way to manage care is to kill the patient"—alerts us to the reciprocal danger of overemphasizing economic definitions. Collaborative discussion and negotiation about quality targets between managed behavioral health care firms and some of the leading academically based clinical programs have started to occur. These have been—and will continue to be—fraught with difficulty, but experience is beginning to emerge that allows cautious optimism (Rogers 1994).

4. *Find new sources of funding for training.* As of mid-1995 only Dr. Pangloss or Pollyanna could be optimistic about finding new funding sources for psychiatric training. The most potent strategy for doing this—the collaborative lobbying approach—has not yet been tried, however.

Academic programs lobby vigorously for continued support for graduate medical education, most notably through Medicare, but the current political climate makes the effectiveness of this effort highly uncertain. Insurers and purchasers are devoting their energy to preventing the cost of education and training from being shifted to them. Medical students are graduating from medical school with high levels of debt and—quite rightly—are not willing to subsidize their own training. No one wants to pay for graduate medical education.

Wise practitioners know that when a clinical situation seems hopeless, convening the involved network of family, friends, and agencies sometimes produces new and useful ideas. Managed behavioral health care companies want to see excellent training continue even though no single company is prepared to make a major unilateral investment in the cost of that training. This seems like an area in which the academic and managed care sectors could usefully join together the involved parties, especially government and large corporations, to seek new approaches to the vexed area of funding.

What Should Academic and Organized Psychiatry Do Now?

Academic psychiatry will have to take the primary initiative for developing the partnerships necessary for robust training in an environment dominated by managed care. The American Association of Directors of Psychiatric Residency Training and the American Association of

Chairmen of Departments of Psychiatry should join together with the American Psychiatric Association Council on Medical Education and Managed Care Committee in outreach to the managed behavioral health care sector on behalf of collaborative promotion of psychiatric training. Doing this will require strategic planning, leadership time, and concerted effort over many years. It is a tremendously demanding project, but it must be done.

To whom should the academic outreachers reach out? This is not a simple question because the national strategy of competition means that managed behavioral health care cannot speak with a single voice. In all likelihood, the best strategy will combine seeking group-to-group partnership with trade associations like the American Managed Behavioral Healthcare Association, the American Association of Health Plans, the HMO Group, and the Institute for Behavioral Healthcare, and at a local level, a series of program-to-program partnerships around particular training ventures.

The group-to-group collaborations could achieve a range of accomplishments. The partners could elaborate an agreed-upon picture of optimal training programs, with the expectation that programs meeting these specifications would be attractive candidates for reimbursement and other forms of support. The managed care sector could recommend a voluntary target, such as "Managed behavioral health care programs should be mindful of a long-term responsibility to support the next generation of clinicians and should ideally devote no less than (X% of revenues) to training purposes." The partners could join with employer groups to lobby for national policies that address training needs. They could jointly investigate and publicize positive examples of program-level collaborations. These ideas merely exemplify the kinds of outcomes collaboration might achieve.

The managed behavioral health care field has been evolving in a fiercely competitive market. Survival and growth have been the predominant corporate strategies for the last decade. The leaders in the field recognize that in the next decade the sector must become as effective at promoting the long-term well-being of the larger health care system as it has been at managing costs. There is no long-term well-being for the mental health field without strong academic psychiatric programs. If academic psychiatry and managed behavioral health care can successfully address the impediments to collaborative action on behalf of their mutual interests, I predict that near the beginning of the twenty-first century we will see examples of substantial new alliances on behalf of education and training.

References

Borus JF: Economics and psychiatric education: the irresistible force meets the moveable object. Harvard Review of Psychiatry 2:15–21, 1994

Frances A: Why a new journal? Journal of Practical Psychiatry and Behavioral Health 1:1, 1995

Gabbard GO: The big chill: the transition from residency to managed care nightmare. Academic Psychiatry 16:119–126, 1992

Kassirer JP: Managed care and the morality of the marketplace. N Engl J Med 333:50–52, 1995

Rako S, Mazer H (eds): Semrad: The Heart of a Therapist. New York, Jason Aronson, 1980

Rogers MC, Snyderman R, Rogers EL: Cultural and organizational implications of academic managed-care networks. N Engl J Med 331: 1374–1377, 1994

Sabin JA: Credo for ethical managed care in mental health practice. Hosp Community Psychiatry 45:859–860, 1994

Sabin JE: The moral myopia of academic psychiatry. Academic Psychiatry 17:175–179, 1993

Schreter RK, Sharfstein SS, Schreter CA (eds): Allies and Adversaries: The Impact of Managed Care on Mental Health Services. Washington, DC, American Psychiatric Press, 1994

CHAPTER EIGHT

Practice Guidelines and Outcomes Management: Future Roles for Psychiatrists

John C. Bartlett, M.D., M.P.H.

> The physician and the patient stand at a strategic point in the general balance of forces in the society of which they are a part.
>
> —Talcott Parsons

> The craftsman is wise in his craft, but, alas, he is all too often willing to pronounce some foolish general judgments.
>
> —Plato

As psychiatry approaches the end of the twentieth century, a century that has witnessed tremendous strides forward both in understanding the causes of many behavioral and emotional disorders and in alleviating much of the attendant suffering and disability, it has much of which to be proud. Yet, rather than enjoying the tremendous progress made to date, psychiatry instead finds itself facing challenges that threaten both its long-standing preeminence within the cadre of mental health practitioners and its very independence as a profession. In the mid-1990s and for the foreseeable future, psychiatrists and their patients increasingly find themselves subjected to concern and skepticism about the value of the activities in which they engage. To some degree, this attention is merely a part of a greater concern on the part of many about the cost of health care. To a large extent, however, psychiatry is singled out for special scrutiny, whether it be expressed through the exponential growth of so-called managed behavioral care techniques or in the seemingly never-ending battle against discrimination directed at both our patients and the resources made available to treat them.

In fact, the organization and delivery of mental health and substance abuse services at the end of the twentieth century is undergoing a series of revolutionary changes. As with most revolutions, these changes are characterized by a break with past approaches and the seemingly inviolable principles that underlie them. It is, in fact, the revolutionary character of these changes that is responsible for much of the turbulence and chaos that psychiatrists are experiencing in their professional lives. At the same time it is also responsible for the inability of old solutions to successfully address the challenges the profession faces; quite simply put, the rules of the game are changing—and changing very rapidly.

Revolution and Roots: Psychiatry as a Scientific Discipline

If there is any comfort that we as psychiatrists can take in the current situation, it must come from the fact that we have successfully faced other revolutions in the past. Yager (1989) points out that in the last 100 years psychiatry has seen at least four revolutions, and in each the psychiatrist was redefined. The first such revolution occurred in the nineteenth century and saw psychiatry move from an earlier tradition of custody to a new one based on humane care. The second began at the end of the nineteenth century and extended well into the present one. This revolution, based on the work of both Freud and his disciples as well as the more somatic therapies such as ECT and medication, saw psychiatry move beyond simple care into concern about causality and even cure. The third revolution began in the 1950s and continued through the 1960s and 1970s and extended the notions of causality and cure from the individual into the community. The fourth revolution began in the 1970s and continues to this day, based largely on major discoveries in the chemistry and biology of behavioral disorders. Yager points out that these revolutions often overlap and that they are shaped by greater economic and social forces. I would maintain, therefore, that we are in the midst of a fifth revolution, one focused on both the cost and the quality of the services and products we provide.

The ultimate aim of this revolution is, at best, to better understand and quantify the value of these products and services; at worst, it represents the latest attempt to discriminate against such services and to severely limit them.

As Yager (1989) has pointed out, in each of these earlier revolutions the role of the psychiatrist was redefined. Yet through all of these redefinitions, one core characteristic remained unchanged; the psychiatrist, with appropriate involvement from the patient, was the sole source of authority and legitimacy in the clinical decision-making process. It was the psychiatrist who differentiated normal from abnormal; it was the psychiatrist who determined the appropriate intervention or set of interventions to restore normality or, at the very least, to mitigate the associated suffering. Throughout all of this, the hallmark of the psychiatrist's role was the independence that he/she was allowed as a professional in the determination and completion of his or her work. Even with the growing emphasis on informed consent and patient autonomy since the 1970s, the relationship between the psychiatrist and the patient was hierarchical between the two and inviolable to the outside world.

Unlike the earlier changes, however, this latest revolution has altered the situation. As the value of the services that mental health and substance abuse practitioners provide has come under increasing scrutiny, the individual psychiatrist has often experienced a significant decrease in his or her degrees of freedom to direct the treatment planning and delivery process. This loss of independence is evident in a number of ways. The most obvious is the ever present case management process to which even the most routine of clinical decisions is now subject. More subtle, perhaps, is the erosion of authority manifested through the ever increasing reduction of benefits available to the individual patient and, therefore, to the treating clinician. At their worst, these reductions completely remove entire levels of care from the decision-making authority of the clinician. The ready justification for this erosion is the need for cost-effectiveness and efficiency in an era of limited health care resources. The effect is to shift the clinician from advocating and allocating in the interests of the patient to managing the interests of not just the patient but also of some larger group or system—a far more complex position. In some cases, that collective represents the employees of one company; in others it may represent entire populations or subpopulations of a state. Ultimately, the important point is that the physician/patient interaction is no longer inviolable and the physician's decision no longer automatically goes unchallenged.

Over the last few years a significant amount of thought and attention has been devoted to the changing role of the psychiatrist in the reorganizing delivery system of the 1990s. A number of conferences and publications (Nadelson and Rabinowitz 1987; Talbott 1989; Yager 1989) have been devoted to such topics as the future of psychiatry as a medical specialty and the future training needs of psychiatrists. All of these efforts have been directed either explicitly or implicitly toward identifying the unique strengths and assets of psychiatry within the range of mental health and substance abuse practitioners, with the ultimate goal of leveraging the resulting opportunities for the benefit of both patients and psychiatrists.

Throughout all of these efforts, the most consistent single theme to be identified is the need for psychiatry to maintain its strong foundations as a scientific discipline, as the branch of medical science that has developed to provide help and treatment for the mentally ill. However, this commitment to helping and treating those who suffer from behavioral and emotional disorders is not enough to distinguish psychiatry from the other professions who minister to the same individuals. Busfield (1986) points out that what ultimately distinguishes the psychiatrist from other helpers of the mentally ill and emotionally disturbed is a further obligation, one that is unique; it is an obligation of method and approach, one that requires the psychiatrist to base his or her actions on medical science and the techniques derived from it. Therefore, scientific knowledge that is based on empirical observation and that conforms to the standards of objectivity that have been developed in the natural sciences should be the foundation of psychiatric care. As a consequence, the concepts, explanations, and treatments offered by psychiatrists can be readily contrasted with the nonscientific, less rational methods of most other mental health and substance abuse practitioners; the role of the psychiatrist is to apply this scientific knowledge in the interests of his or her individual patients.

It is essential to point out, however, that in all this discussion of the scientific foundations of psychiatry, the principles and processes involved are not only chemical, physical, or biological ones. To this extent it is important to differentiate the scientific basis of psychiatry from the so-called medical model, which is far more limited in scope. According to Busfield (1986), "this concentration on physical processes has become the virtual hallmark of medicine and the terms medical and physical are at times used synonymously, as in the use of the term 'medical model,' to refer to the assumption that mental illness can be explained, understood, and treated in physical terms" (p. 26). Far from restricting its interests to the purely physical, however, psychiatry, because of the very special nature of the illnesses and conditions it seeks to treat, must bring its scientific perspective and approach to bear on a much wider range of phenomena, including not merely the biological but also the psychological and the social. Psychiatry, then, differs from most of the rest of medicine in openly addressing a broader range of content; it must differ from the other mental health and substance professions by having a greater precision and objectivity of process.

This breadth of content and depth of approach bode well for psychiatry to be at the center of any reorganized delivery system for mental health and substance abuse. Many even say that the central role of psychiatry in diagnosis, treatment planning, and treatment follow-up will position psychiatry as the principal arbiter of quality in the future. Others, however, are not so sure. They rightly point out that psychiatry, particularly in clinical practice, still has far to go in its efforts to become truly science based and therefore distinct from the other mental health professions. Yager (1989) outlines the challenges facing psychiatric science in areas such as developing reliable and valid nosologies and measuring and relating outcomes to treatment, among others.

Revolution in the Marketplace: The Challenge of Value

These challenges to our scientific foundations allow the marketplace to question our authority to be the sole judge of quality because they undercut our ability to be consistent in our definitions, our models, and our treatments. And this lack of consistency is at the core of the marketplace's skepticism about psychiatry. In fact, it is this very lack of consistency in both model and approach, coupled with an increased awareness of cost, that has provided the opportunity for the development and growth of managed approaches to the delivery of mental health and substance abuse care. It is a fallacy to see the success of the managed behavioral care industry as arising purely from a concern for cost containment. Instead, it has developed out of questions about the value of the services provided. These questions most often take the form of concerns about the level of quality and results generated for the level of dollars spent.

Managed behavioral care has attempted to address this marketplace concern about value by managing benefits through the determination of the medical appropriateness of treatment plans. In and of itself there is nothing revolutionary about this approach; in fact, it merely represents the extension of tools and techniques from the management of medical and surgical care, such as utilization review and case management. What has been revolutionary and, in fact, caused most of the uproar and concern among clinicians has been the fact that managed care has restricted the wide range of what constitutes medically appropriate care that was tolerated in the past. By so doing it has attempted to squarely confront what one author (Giles 1991) has called the "equivalency of therapies" myth. From a strategic point of view, therefore, managed care represents a very successful attempt to reduce variability in the treatment of mental health and substance abuse disorders. It has attempted to drive this reduction in variability in the direction of cost-effectiveness, guided to the greatest extent possible by the available clinical and health services research and applicable clinical experience. However, to the extent that there are gaps in the science concerning comparative cost effectiveness of treatments for specific conditions (and there are many), we have left the door open for concern about cost alone to be the determinant of the types and amounts of favored care.

But in limiting the range of so-called medically appropriate and therefore reimbursable treatments, what effect has managed care had on the quality of the care provided? In an era when the direct costs of care can be reduced 20%, 30%, even 40% or more, this should become an important concern. In addressing this concern, however, a crucial point to understand is that managed care's attempts to drive a less variable, more consistent approach to treatment does not necessarily threaten quality at all; in fact, the very opposite may be true. This is because the payers in their own areas of business have moved beyond the subjective, ill-defined kind of quality known only to a small group of insiders (the quality model that has traditionally been employed in health care) to a more objective, measurable, and ultimately improvable type of quality. In this regard, managed care is being shaped by significant changes in the approach to the definition and demonstration of quality that are currently underway in many areas of American business. Whether these changes are called total quality management or continuous quality improvement or something else, the goal of the effort is the measurement of demonstrable improvement in quality over time, and the prophets, such as Deming and Juran, most often have engineering backgrounds.

Under this approach to quality, the process is one of defining objective standards and then managing the variation around these standards. The goal is not mindless uniformity; it is instead the reduction of complexity, waste, and rework. These goals are achieved through the collection and analysis of data produced throughout the implementation of the specified process; the results of this analysis are used to identify opportunities to improve the process and therefore ultimately the results it is capable of delivering. A key point to realize is that under this rubric any unexplained and unmanaged variability represents a potential threat to quality; although not necessarily bad in and of itself, such unexplained variability is seen as inherently problematic, wasteful, and inefficient.

Value and Science: The New Approach to Quality

Berwick and his coauthors (1990) have developed 10 core principles of this new approach to quality and its application in the organization and delivery of health care. Although all 10 principles are essential to a full understanding of the approach, of particular interest in the context of the foregoing discussion are the fifth principle—*understanding the variability of processes is a key to improving quality*—and the seventh principle—*the modern approach to quality is thoroughly grounded in scientific and statistical thinking*. What Berwick and others are in essence describing is a fundamental and complete shift in the paradigm that governs the definition and appreciation of quality in health care. In fact, the quality paradigm is changing (and to a large extent has already changed) from that of the artisan, where quality was defined in idiosyncratic, individual, and often subjective ways, to that of the engineer, where it is measured against objective standards and defined by the degree of conformance to these standards. This development in no way preempts what has traditionally been considered to be the art of clinical practice; it merely places that art at the level of the individual patient and in the context of the larger delivery system.

For a number of years, many psychiatric leaders have either been aware of or intuitively responding to this shift. Fully five years ago Herb Pardes identified the absence of any broad consensus in the field of psychiatry as a problem for the profession (Talbott 1989). In fact, the primary recommendation of a 1987 conference on the future of psychiatry sponsored by the American Psychiatric Association and attended by an extensive representation of psychiatric leaders was the following: *Because the overarching issue for the future will be the quality of care provided to our patients, quality of care must be ensured through increased and improved efforts to set and enforce standards* (Talbott 1989). Although the emphasis on enforcement is not entirely in keeping with the principles of quality improvement, the basic recognition and endorsement of the central role of standards in the definition and evaluation of quality in psychiatric practice is. Even psychiatrists in training recognize the lack of consensus within the field and respond negatively to it; in their 1986–1987 survey of PGY-4 residents, Weissman and Bashook found no consistent patterns of experience shared by a majority of trainees, even in the area of long-term psychotherapy. In describing their findings, the authors point out a number of the difficulties caused by the lack of a standardized foundation for the profession (Nadelson and Rabinowitz 1987).

In light of the historical absence of broadly accepted standards of psychiatric quality, one might well ask if this change in quality paradigms is really such a good thing. This question can and should be debated, but two points must be considered in any such discussion. The first, which has already been made, is that this very lack of standardization and consensus about appropriate care has prevented the marketplace from developing any consistent impression of the quality of our work as psychiatrists. In fact, this very lack of standards has directly caused the marketplace's concern about the value of mental health and substance abuse care. This in turn has led many clinicians to feel that they are caught between the Scylla of benefit restrictions and the Charybdis of managed care. The second point is that, whether good or bad, the paradigm shift has already begun and, in fact, now has sufficient momentum to be all but inevitable. The "industrialization" of health care is every day more of a reality, and the associated calls for demonstrable value and quality, not just cost savings, are everywhere. Furthermore, when one considers that the organization and delivery of health care goods and services constitute some 15% of our gross domestic product, this transition from a "cottage industry" to a more sophisticated form of oversight and management seems not just inevitable but perhaps even long overdue.

The Industrialization of Behavioral Health Care

In light of the current situation, then, it is perhaps instructive to examine similar shifts that have taken place in other fields, where traditional methods of accomplishing work have been replaced. One powerful such example is that of the mechanization of many aspects of production that took place in Europe and the Americas during the eighteenth and nineteenth centuries, the so-called Industrial Revolution. In fact, the Industrial Revolution is often represented as a matter of direct and open conflict between industry, with its appetite for quantity and uniformity, on the one hand, and craft, with its fascination with "quality" and individuality, on the other. As Lucie-Smith (1981) points out, however, this depiction of a strict and inseparable division between industry and craft is a gross oversimplification, and, in fact, the Industrial Revolution arose from the combination of many factors and forces, some economic, some esthetic, some purely social and egalitarian. The industrialization of any craft is far from a simple matter, either in process, content, or result, and is always difficult to reduce to a simple matter of good or bad.

Perhaps the best example given by Lucie-Smith is that of the industrialization of the production of pottery in England during the mid-eighteenth century. Prior to this time pottery was largely a craft, with each pot being made mostly by hand, with the aid of simple tools and techniques such as the potter's wheel and the kiln. The quality and quantity of production was left entirely to the judgment and skill of the individual potter. However, as both commerce and the standard of living throughout England increased with the establishment and growth of the empire, the potter's craft came under increasing pressure to produce both greater quantities as well as greater quality. Each step of the potter's process, therefore, was exposed to continual demand for improvement in order to increase production to meet growing demand. Moreover, as classicism, with its idealization of the forms of ancient Greece and Rome, became the standard of quality, it often proved to be too difficult for the average craftsperson to master.

Into this situation of some turmoil and great opportunity entered Josiah Wedgewood. An artisan and entrepreneur of great energy and skill, Wedgewood developed standardized forms and molds that successfully captured (and, in fact, even defined) classical taste in a style of china called Queen's ware. In addition, in his use of methods and materials for production, he relentlessly pursued organization, rationalization, and standardization. By the end of his career, the simple craft shop that at first had employed only Wedgewood and a handful of apprentices had become a huge factory with scores of buildings requiring a canal for transport of finished goods to markets all over the world. As Lucie-Smith points out, the real significance of Queen's ware arose not from the fact that the Empress Catherine of Russia ordered a 952-piece set for her imperial court. Rather, through innovative standards of quality and production, Josiah Wedgewood made fine tableware of absolutely even and reliable quality available to a much larger range of customers than ever before!

This story and others like it from the history of industry undercut the largely romantic notion that industrialization represents the demise of quality. Although it may be true that individuality is reduced with the application of standardized forms and processes, production and availability can be greatly increased, costs can be contained and even reduced, and quality can be defined, demonstrated, and improved. All of these sound like appropriate and even laudable goals for psychiatry in an era of increasing need and decreasing resources. What is involved here again, however, is an acceptance of a different model of quality than has traditionally held sway in health care, and, most importantly, an appreciation of the central role of objective, documented standards under this new model. In fact, the whole concept of quality improvement involves a change in the theoretical role of standards, from seeing them as thresholds ("everything above is OK") to establishing them as ideals. Under this rubric the goal of quality efforts becomes focused not on using standards as tools to cull "bad apples" but rather on monitoring, analyzing, and minimizing variation around them. Standards become rallying points, if you will, positions or goals that legitimately require us to measure all else against them.

Guidelines and Outcomes: The New Tools of Psychiatric Science

In applying this new quality paradigm to the organization and delivery of psychiatric services, the appropriate role of practice guidelines becomes clear. Practice guidelines (and other forms of clinical standards, such as level of care guidelines) are potential tools for reducing the variation in clinical practice and in so doing are central to the definition and demonstration of quality. They do so by documenting with the greatest specificity possible the processes of care that should be adopted in any given clinical situation. Two key points emerge from this statement. The first is that, for practice guidelines to serve as standards and ideals, they must derive their authority from legitimate and recognized sources. In clinical areas we must all become comfortable with and supportive of the notion that the major source of legitimacy must be scientifically sound clinical and health services research. Fred Goodwin, in addressing a major meeting of the managed behavioral care industry in 1991, clearly echoed this sentiment by saying "We can as a society no longer afford to fund the idiosyncratic judgment of individual clinicians. Reimbursement must be driven by the research."

In underscoring the central role that scientifically sound research must play in the determination of appropriate care (and therefore in the development of practice guidelines, which document these determinations in readily accessible formats), it is important also to recognize the need for flexibility and discretion in the application of these guidelines to the treatment of individual patients. Given the current state of knowledge in our field and the basic and very real differences between the environments in which sound efficacy research is conducted and in which most patient care is delivered, guidelines should be seen as at most directing, not controlling, clinical practice. They are basically a means of informing the clinical judgment of clinicians by distilling current knowledge and making explicit current "best practices." In saying this it becomes important to recognize that clinical judgment has two distinct components. According to Feinstein (1967), the first is the therapeutic component, that which addresses the question "What is the best treatment for this disorder?" The second is the environmental, which asks the separate question "What is the best way to deliver that treatment to this patient?" Feinstein rightfully points out that, whereas the environmental component of clinical judgment is so complex so as to be incapable of any meaningful empirical analysis and, in fact, represents the art of clinical practice, the therapeutic component is entirely subject to empirical investigation and therefore must be based in sound science. It becomes clear, then, that in developing an appropriate role for practice guidelines in the direction of clinical practice, it is essential to see them as addressing the therapeutic component of clinical judgment, the part that lies rightfully in the realm of empirical investigation. On the other hand, the environmental component dictates flexibility in their application to individual patients and therefore represents what has traditionally been called the art of clinical practice.

The second key point that emerges from our new understanding of practice guidelines as standards around which clinical practice can be centered is that they must be collaboratively produced, documented in explicit and accessible formats, and ultimately be as specific as possible if they are to serve as tools to reduce variation. It should be self-evident that, in order to serve as rallying points, guidelines must represent a consensus of both the most empirically informed and clinically sensitive thinking available at any given time. While comprehensive and detailed reviews of the clinical and health services research literature must be the foundation of their development, discussion and, ultimately, reasoned compromise will most likely always be involved in their production, if for no other reason than that no individual research study is "perfect," and therefore all are open to differing interpretations.

And again, in order to serve as rallying points, guidelines must be accessible, useable, and available. The question of accessibility directly addresses the question of what value guidelines ultimately hold for the practicing clinician and his or her patient. After all, if guidelines merely reflect the knowledge that is already contained in the scientific literature, what purpose do they serve? The answer to this question lies in considering the premise underlying it, which is that the knowledge base contained in the scientific literature is routinely reflected in clinical practice. As Goodwin pointed out some years ago in the remarks cited earlier, this application of research-based knowledge is all too infrequently seen in clinical practice. In turn, this situation reflects poorly on the scientific foundations of psychiatry that, as has already been pointed out, should serve to distinguish us from other mental health and substance abuse professionals. The reasons for this failure of contemporary scientific knowledge to be reflected in much of clinical practice can and should be debated; the important point for this discussion is that practice guidelines, appropriately developed and presented, can be important tools for communicating the consensus of experts as to what the current state of knowledge is. Furthermore, for this reason guidelines should be as specific and structured as possible. Rather than narratives that dance around controversial areas of the current state of knowledge (or, even worse, that represent purely political positions or narrow guild interests), they should be structured so as to delineate clear and actionable positions for the practicing clinician. The agency for Healthcare Policy and Research recognizes the importance of this point by including a set of process maps in its quick reference guides for clinicians, along with more encyclopedic narrative reviews of the salient literature. Psychiatry should do the same with its practice guidelines. The crucial point here is that the flexibility essential to the accommodation of sound clinical judgment should not be achieved through the narrative formatting of guidelines, which will only continue to promote subjectivity in our clinical work and prevent any adequate definition or demonstration of quality. Instead, the requisite flexibility should be achieved through their sensitive implementation, with allowance for and monitoring of those patient-specific indicators that drive the need for exceptions to the standards. In short, the need for specificity in documentation and flexibility in implementation of practice guidelines is essential for the realization of their potential to address variability in clinical practice because one can begin to measure their impact and even their acceptability in practice only through this approach.

With specific, documented guidelines in place that represent consensus opinion about the current state of knowledge, psychiatry will have taken a major step forward in addressing the wide variability in our field. Yet a greater question remains: "Are our consensus standards in fact correct?" In producing documented clinical guidelines and standards, have we in fact controlled variation around a position that reflects some higher truth and therefore has a legitimate claim to serve as an ideal? After all, consensus standards, even ones driven by a reasoned analysis of the available empirical evidence, still represent at best a distillation of the current state of knowledge at any given time. And knowledge, in turn, can change, either incrementally, through expansion of current beliefs, or exponentially, through the generation and adoption of entirely new intellectual models or paradigms (Kuhn 1962). For example, the consensus judgment of physicians about ether anesthesia before 1846 may well have considered it the devil's work. In our own field, consider how our understanding of and approach to treatment of such conditions as obsessive-compulsive disorder has changed markedly over the last decade. The challenge here is that consensus, by definition, limits variability and may even ultimately frustrate efforts to develop new and better ways of caring for patients. Therefore, some means of establishing the validity (or lack thereof) of our consensus positions is clearly needed—some capability to empirically determine whether they are indeed valid standards of quality.

I believe that, in the near term, the only truly effective means of demonstrating quality in mental health and substance abuse care is through the measurement of outcomes. Why is this so? After all, outcomes is only one of the three widely accepted parameters of clinical quality first developed by Avedis Donabedian (Donabedian 1982); the others are structure and process. Here again it is the wide variability in both model and approach found today in clinical practice that minimizes the utility of structure and process measures of quality in our field. Each model and approach has its own hallowed approaches, often widely different and equally often the product of opinion rather than science. These differences make the development of meaningful standards based on structure or process a difficult, if not a futile, task. Just attempt to envision any set of meaningful (and, more importantly, manageable) standards developed by a mix of psychoanalytically oriented therapists, biologically oriented psychiatrists, and behaviorists; now consider that even this mix is at best a narrow reflection of prevailing models and approaches to treatment within many of our areas of clinical practice.

The solution to the quality dilemma created by the current range of treatment models is to measure the results of their application—their outcomes, if you will. With such a process in place, the analysis of the results can inform our explorations of treatment structure and process; we will have in place a feedback loop, in effect, that will allow for not just the measurement but also over time the demonstrable improvement of our clinical tools and techniques. It should be clear from these statements that what is called for is not simply research into the outcomes of the care we provide, but rather the use of this information in an ongoing and systematic way to inform and ultimately to guide management decisions at both the delivery system and the individual patient level. Outcomes research, whether it examines questions of efficacy, effectiveness, or something else, is an academic discipline most often conducted in the milieu of the university or policy institute. Outcomes management, on the other hand, is a management tool that builds on the methodologies developed in the academic setting to address a wide range of clinical and administrative questions. Although outcomes management programs can be built around individual studies, the state of the art in outcomes management approaches is that of the outcomes system. In contrast to a single study, a biopsy, if you will, the results of which become outmoded as soon as they are used to make any improvements in care, an outcomes system represents an ongoing management process designed to collect sound data about a wide variety of outcomes of interest, provide for its ongoing aggregation and analysis, and, most importantly, feed this information to a variety of end users for their consideration and action. It should be obvious to even the casual observer that contemporary managed behavioral care organizations perform many, but not all, of these key functions. As a part of their activities, they routinely collect data about a variety of areas of central importance to such an outcomes management approach. These areas include financial, benefit design, demographic, and clinical data, among others.

The first shortcoming is that, to date, the scientific challenges of collecting sound data about outcome domains of interest have most often not been addressed. These challenges include such areas as collecting clinical data in structured formats in order to aggregate it into large databases, establishing the reliability and validity of the data collected, determining the baseline status of patients prior to treatment in order to quantify posttreatment improvements, and, finally, recognizing the need for adequate data about case-mix factors in order to examine differential treatment effects. The true promise of managed care, therefore, lies in its largely unrealized potential to generate huge databases about clinical outcomes and to link these databases to others, such as financial, benefit design, utilization, and even theoretically payer-based data (e.g., medical/surgical claims, absenteeism, and productivity). This linkage would in turn allow the exploration of such crucial policy issues as the cost-effectiveness of mental health and substance abuse care from not simply a paid claims point of view but, more importantly, from a larger benefit systems frame of reference. With this kind of information about not just the direct costs of providing appropriate mental health and addictive disorders care but, more importantly, the quality and indirect cost savings associated with this care, we as psychiatrists would be better able to demonstrate the value of our efforts.

Industrialization as Opportunity

Although the organizational challenges involved in realizing such a vision are significant, the potential value to all of the various stakeholders in the current debate about the value of mental health and substance abuse care is considerable. Once we utilize organized delivery systems that routinely employ explicit practice guidelines to reduce variability in practice and to track and analyze the outcomes of the application of those guidelines, we will have taken a major step forward in establishing the true value of the clinical services and programs we provide as psychiatrists. More importantly, by adopting a more structured and quantitative approach to the measurement and improvement of clinical quality, we will reinforce our key position as the providers of mental health and substance abuse services with firm and long-standing foundations in empirical science. One need only consider the benefits that have accrued to psychiatry through the generation of structured, explicit diagnostic criteria, which are now the standard of diagnosis for all disciplines and entities. In a similar fashion, the generation of structured and explicit treatment planning and monitoring criteria (e.g., practice guidelines and outcomes management systems) will only enhance our stature and our influence. By accepting that scientific psychiatry need not be limited to the biological sciences but can easily embrace and profit from the knowledge base of the social and even the engineering sciences, we can easily establish a central role for both practice guidelines and outcomes management as important tools of the psychiatrist of the future. In the hands of tomorrow's psychiatrists, structure and quality will not be enemies; indeed, they will be allies.

References

Berwick D, Godfrey A, Roessner J: Curing Health Care: New Strategies for Quality Improvement. San Francisco, CA, Jossey-Bass, 1990
Busfield J: Managing Madness: Changing Ideas and Practice. London, Hutchinson, 1986
Donabedian A: Explorations in Quality Assessment and Monitoring. Ann Arbor, MI, Health Administration Press, 1982

Feinstein A: Clinical Judgment. Baltimore, MD, Williams & Wilkins, 1967
Field M, Lohr K: Guidelines for Clinical Practice: From Development to Use. Washington, DC, National Academy Press, 1992
Giles T: Managed mental health care and effective psychotherapy. J Behav Ther Exp Psychiatry 22:83–86, 1991
Kuhn T: The Structure of Scientific Revolutions. Chicago, IL, University of Chicago Press, 1962
Lucie-Smith E: The Story of Craft: The Craftsman's Role in Society. Ithaca, NY, Cornell University Press, 1981
Nadelson C, Rabinowitz C (eds): Training Psychiatrists for the '90s: Issues and Recommendations. Washington, DC, American Psychiatric Press, 1987
Talbott J (ed): Future Directions for Psychiatry. Washington, DC, American Psychiatric Press, 1989
Yager J (ed): The Future of Psychiatry as a Medical Specialty. Washington, DC, American Psychiatric Press, 1989

CHAPTER NINE

The Physician-Patient Relationship in a Managed Care Setting: Informed Consent, Confidentiality, and Trust

Elaine M. Buzzinotti, J.D.
Loren H. Roth, M.D., M.P.H.
Thomas L. Horn, M.D.

> In the covenant with our patients we find our professional identity and ethics.
>
> —Webb 1989

Health care reform with its focus on managed care and competition raises a number of questions about the role of the physician in the various service delivery models. Conflicts of interest, financial and otherwise, threaten the integrity of the traditional physician-patient relationship. Increasingly, provider "networks" are replacing the single practitioner in many areas of medicine. This chapter examines the evolution of the doctor-patient relationship in the context of health care reform, with an emphasis on psychiatry. Following an overview of the history of the physician-patient relationship and its connection with the doctrines of confidentiality and informed consent, the authors provide a synopsis of managed care and discuss the draft Report of the Council on Ethical and Judicial Affairs (CEJA) of the American Medical Association. The authors summarize the report's recommendations that the medical profession, along with society, respond affirmatively to the challenges of managed care in ways that 1) prioritize patient needs in maintaining the integrity of the physician-patient relationship and 2) preserve the fundamental duty of physicians as patient advocates. The authors posit that, under the "old ethics," the physician's core conflict was the tension between physician paternalism and patient autonomy, whereas, under the "new ethics," which is driven in part by managed care practices, the conflict is one of physician indifference versus patient advocacy (American Medical Association 1994).

The Physician-Patient Relationship: Two Models of Moral Responsibility

Ethical aspects of the physician-patient relationship have historically focused on the moral responsibility of the individual physician to his or her individual patient. In so doing, the traditional model of the physician-patient relationship encouraged a view of the patient as a passive participant in a two-party, doctor-patient dyad (Beauchamp and McCullough 1984). In this model, "medicine," as represented in the person of the physician, determines the patient's best interests by becoming the primary, if not sole, determiner of the intervention(s). As set forth in the Hippocratic oath, the physician is obligated to benefit the sick and avoid harm and injustice (Beauchamp and McCullough 1984). Thus, in the traditional doctor-patient model, the principle of beneficence is the fundamental moral principle from which the physician's moral obligations and virtues are derived (Beauchamp and McCullough 1984). Proponents of this model emphasize the advantages of the physician-as-fiduciary in determining the best interests of the patient. Notwithstanding some of the benefits that can be derived from benign paternalism, a strict construction of this model can serve to place the patient in a highly dependent and vulnerable position. With power and decision making held almost exclusively by the physician, a strict or total adherence to the beneficence model can compromise patient autonomy and freedom of choice.

An alternative model of moral responsibility for physicians that evolved from the doctrine of informed consent (discussed in the next section) is the autonomy model. In this model, the values and beliefs of the patient (as opposed to the physician) are given primary moral consideration. Thus, if the adult rational patient's values directly conflict with medicine's values, it is the fundamental responsibility of the physician to "respect and facilitate a patient's self-determination in making decisions about his or her medical fate" (Beauchamp and McCullough 1984). In this model, the primary, if not sole, fundamental moral principle is the respect for autonomy, from which the physician's moral obligations are derived (Beauchamp and McCullough 1984). In the autonomy model, the physician may not presume to independently pursue the best interests of the patient as medicine alone would define them. Rather, the model requires respect for patients' decisions in all matters pursuant to their medical care. A strict construction of this model views the physician-patient relationship as a partnership of "equal standing" with an equally shared balance of power in terms of medical decision making, notwithstanding the parties' different motivations and knowledge bases.

There is a general theoretical concurrence that the successful resolution of medical-ethical issues in the physician-patient relationship is best accomplished by balancing the beneficent with the autonomy models to meet the individual needs of patients. As we will argue, managed care delivery systems are optimally therapeutic when ethical responsibilities attach to all participating parties (i.e., the plan itself, the physician participant, and the patient consumer).

Informed Consent

As first articulated by the courts, the doctrine of informed consent required physicians to provide thorough explanations to patients about proposed specific treatments or procedures so that patients would have adequate information with which to voluntarily provide or refuse consent (Salgo v Leland Stanford Junior University Board of Trustees 1957). In the early developmental period of this legal doctrine, the substance of the disclosure made to patients was primarily determined by medical judgment. Thus, "[t]he duty of the physician to disclose ... is limited to those disclosures which a reasonable medical practitioner would make under the same or similar circumstances" (Natansan v Kline 1960). This became known as the professional standard of disclosure, and by its terms, what—if anything—was disclosed was what the physician determined to be in the patient's best interest. Thus, although the patient was deemed to be entitled to certain information, the professional standard of disclosure model enabled the physician to apply beneficent principles with regard to what in fact was disclosed (Appelbaum et al. 1987).

As the doctrine of informed consent evolved, it was subsequently extended to require additional disclosure to patients. Such disclosures included additional information about any proposed treatments or procedures and their related risks and benefits; available alternatives to the proposed treatment or procedures were also required.

The expansion of the doctrine of informed consent paralleled the evolution of the doctor-patient relationship in the direction of self-determination and autonomy. An alternative to the professional standard of disclosure, the "materiality," or "patient-centered" standard, was the result. Under the terms of this standard, the obligation of the physician to disclose became one of what a "reasonable person" would want to know about a procedure or treatment before consenting to it (Canterbury v Spence 1972). Both the professional and patient-centered standards of review are utilized today, and the standard in use in a particular jurisdiction varies according to state law. Not only is the debate over the preferred standard unresolved, but to further complicate matters, some courts have imposed components of the two standards of disclosure, forming a "hybrid" standard. Under such a standard, liability can be imposed if a physician withholds information that under *either* a professional standard *or* a patient-centered standard would be deemed to warrant disclosure (Appelbaum et al. 1987). As discussed in the section on managed care and informed consent, a variation on the hybrid standard is recommended for adoption in managed care delivery systems.

Notwithstanding what standard of review is employed, there is also a lack of professional consensus as to the content of what should be disclosed. At common law, the minimum elements of disclosure for informed consent include 1) the nature and purpose of the proposed procedure or treatment; 2) risks, including an estimate of "material," "substantial," "probable," or "significant"; 3) anticipated benefits or probability of success; and 4) the availability of other options or alternatives (Appelbaum et al. 1987). The latter includes the option of no treatment (Appelbaum et al. 1987), which is especially important in psychiatry. For example, a psychiatrist should review, at a minimum, the consequences of a no-treatment choice in terms of the patient's risk of relapse, including the likelihood for more aggressive and/or restrictive treatment in the absence of compliance with the proposed treatment (Klerman et al. 1986). As we will discuss, the process and content of disclosure when viewed in the context of managed care is critical to the preservation of a viable and therapeutic doctor-patient relationship.

For consent to be informed, it needs to be voluntarily made and understood by a competent patient. The law presumes capacity and understanding. However, these areas can be especially difficult to determine in psychiatry. Generally, a patient demonstrates capacity upon a manifestation of an appreciation of the nature, extent, and probable consequences of the proposed intervention (Appelbaum et al. 1987). The degree of complexity of the treatment and its consequences, in addition to the patient's mental status at the time consent is being sought, need to be considered when determining capacity. Understanding can be difficult to assess in psychiatry, but all efforts should be made to assess patient understanding of treatment options. In addition to consideration of the complexity of the proposed treatment, the patient's present mental status and premorbid level of functioning should factor into assessments of understanding and true voluntariness.

There are four major exceptions to informed consent: 1) emergency, 2) incapacity, 3) therapeutic privilege, and 4) waiver (Appelbaum et al. 1987).

A long-standing tradition in medical practice, with origins in common law, holds that consent need not be obtained in medical emergencies. If informed consent is withheld due to an emergency, it should be because the time involved in making the disclosure and obtaining a patient's informed decision would be detrimental to a compelling medical interest of the patient (Appelbaum et al. 1987). The urgency of a situation is determined primarily by the potential consequences to the patient caused by delay in the rendition of treatment or failure to render any treatment at all (Appelbaum et al. 1987). Definitions of emergency range from those submitted by rights advocates, who propose a narrow construction (one that would promote the most autonomy in decision making), to those offered by caregivers, physicians in particular, who propose a broader interpretation in order to minimize the possibility of causing irreparable harm to the patient or others.

Incapacity is another exception to the physician's duty to provide informed consent. To the extent that a patient's incapacity involves decision making pursuant to his or her medical care, the incapacitated patient cannot provide informed consent for such care. In psychiatry, capacity may be in flux, and determination of capacity more difficult and subject to change. A patient's capacity can be general or specific. If the patient is deemed to be generally incapacitated, then the physician's duties of disclosure and consent are suspended for all intent and purposes (Appelbaum et al. 1987). If the patient is deemed to be generally competent, which is the legal presumption, physicians are obligated to attempt disclosure. A patient may be deemed to be incapacitated in a particular area only after disclosure and an attempt to obtain consent have been initiated. As Appelbaum points out, the incapacity exception differs from the other exceptions to the requirement of obtaining informed consent, in that the requirement is not negated, but rather changed in form. That is, a substitute decision maker to provide such consent is required (Appelbaum and Gutheil 1991).

Therapeutic privilege is the third exception to informed consent. The physician is suspended from providing informed consent pursuant to the nature of a patient's condition and proposed treatment if, in the physician's opinion, the information to be conveyed would in itself be so damaging to the patient that disclosure would be antitherapeutic (Appelbaum and Gutheil 1991).

Finally, informed consent need not be provided to patients who do not want it, who have asked not to receive it, or who request an abbreviated form of disclosure. This is the waiver exception, which brings the process of self-determination and autonomous decision making full circle. In exercising this exception, it is imperative that patients affirmatively indicate such a preference to the physician, as opposed to the physician's making an independent determination not to inform as a function of physician avoidance or refusal to so engage the patient. Informed consent is an ethical imperative of the physician (Klerman et al. 1986), and as with the construct of confidentiality in the context of the physician-patient privilege, ownership of waiver vests with the patient—not the physician.

Confidentiality

Article nine of the AMA Principles of Medical Ethics sets forth the standards of the physician's ethical obligation of confidentiality:

> A physician may not reveal the confidences entrusted to him in the course of medical attendance; or the deficiencies he may observe in the character of patients, unless it becomes necessary to protect the welfare of the individual or community. (American Medical Association 1984)

Traditionally, the application of confidentiality in a health care setting refers to patients' rightful expectations that medical records and related communications pursuant to their status of health will be treated confidentially by health care providers. Subject to certain exceptions, confidentiality of health-related information applies to all areas of medicine, but additional protection is afforded mental health information. In fact, 11 of the annotations attached to the AMA principles and specifically applicable to psychiatry directly address issues of confidentiality (Webb 1989). The legal sources of such treatment are found in federal and state constitutional privacy rights; federal and state laws and regulations governing confidentiality of mental health record information; and state laws pursuant to the physician-patient privilege. The justifications for the "superconfidential" treatment of psychiatric information are multifold. First, confidentiality is critical in psychiatry as it is intrinsic to the formation of a therapeutic relationship. Confidentiality is the very foundation of the doctor-patient relationship and affirms and protects the fundamental value of personal privacy. In turn, such assurance and expectation encourage persons who need professional assistance to seek it voluntarily, while facilitating the development of the trust and confidence essential for therapeutic intervention. Confidentiality is desirable because it also provides protection against the socially and/or economically stigmatizing consequences of help-seeking behavior (e.g., a patient is forced into early retirement from a job or denied adequate housing secondary to receiving psychiatric assistance). Finally, confidentiality is desirable in that it promotes patient self-determination and autonomy in decision making. Ownership of this privilege ostensibly vests solely with the patient. However, as discussed later on, pursuant to the written or unwritten terms of a health plan agreement related to the need to review extensive clinical data as a precondition of payment, the plan can become a constructive co-owner of the privilege. Put another way, the patient can be essentially precluded from independent exercise of the privilege by the threat or actual denial of benefits.

A generally recognized exception to the requirement of patient consent for the release of confidential information is the presence of third-party payers for reimbursement purposes. However, this exception is usually narrowly defined by regulation pursuant to confidentiality provisions of state mental health statutes to include a minimum of information. Such regulations were drafted at a time when fee-for-service compensation plans and related retrospective utilization review prevailed and there was no need for such extensive information as requested by managed care entities for precertification and concurrent review purposes.

As we will discuss later on, managed care raises a host of confidentiality-related issues, including those concerning how to respond to a growing number of individuals in the network claiming a medically based "need to know," which is another generally recognized exception to patient consent. This exception has traditionally been restricted to those professionals who are actively engaged in the consultation, diagnoses, and/or treatment of the patient (Feldman and Fitzpatrick 1992).

There are also confidentiality issues associated with electronic data systems (EDS) and "information superhighways," as managed care networks increasingly turn to such technology for storage and transmission of health information.

Managed Care and the Practice of Medicine

There has been a growing concern among Americans over the rising cost of health care for some time. This concern has now culminated in a national debate about how such costs may best be contained. One solution is managed care. In its most basic form, managed care refers to those interventions in the delivery and financing of health care that are intended to eliminate unnecessary and inappropriate care and, by so doing, reduce costs (Congressional Budget Office 1992). Studies have supported a pattern of economic loss pursuant to traditional fee-for-service health care delivery and thus reinforced the need for cost containment (Morreim 1991). Toward this end, managed care has been advocated since the 1970s, and the concept has been rapidly evolving since then. There are various delivery models of service provision among what is generally subsumed under managed care. The common element shared among all such approaches is the prospective or concurrent review of care provided to individual patients, with the power to deny payment for care deemed to be not medically necessary or cost effective. This is in contrast to the retrospective review primarily associated with traditional fee-for-service delivery models.

The major aspects of managed care include the following (Congressional Budget Office 1992):

1. Reviewing and intervening in decisions about providing health services
2. Establishing a network of providers and then requiring or influencing patients to use those providers
3. Negotiating different payment terms with providers

Managed care practices are not new. Precursors to the present-day application of managed care include the following methods of restricting health care expenditures: 1) state and federal certificates of need (CON) requirements; 2) physician review organizations (PROs), which are utilization review (UR) committees prescribed by the Health Care Finance Administration (HCFA); and 3) diagnostic related groupings (DRGs), a prospective method of containing nonpsychiatric inpatient hospitalization costs by diagnostic classification. However, individually and collectively, these methods have not adequately contained rising health care costs.

Today, management of care occurs within essentially all health care payment systems. In traditional indemnity programs, in which patients choose their providers, who are in turn reimbursed on a fee-for-service basis, precertification for admission and/or treatment authorization is frequently mandated. Public health insurance programs (e.g., Medicare and Medicaid) are also rapidly moving in the direction of managed care methodologies of cost containment.

In health maintenance organizations (HMOs), insurance coverage is combined with an internal delivery system, and services are covered only when the beneficiary uses the organization's delivery system (Congressional Budget Office 1992). In an HMO, care is delivered by a preset group of providers for a fixed annual fee. Gatekeepers, usually in the form of primary medical practitioners, are designated to serve in a prescreening role. Selection of treatment modalities is governed by uniform protocols or guidelines that restrict provider discretion (Appelbaum 1993). HMO providers' compensation is affected by their cost-controlling abilities, either directly, through bonuses or penalties, or indirectly, through payments linked to the overall profit of the organization (Appelbaum 1993).

In contrast to an HMO, a preferred provider organization (PPO) contracts with an insurance company or employer to arrange a network or panel of providers whose services are offered to beneficiaries of the insurance plan or members of the employment group. In PPOs patients are limited to determined panels of providers, or they are offered an economic incentive to select a provider from the panel (Appelbaum 1993).

Within HMO and PPO models, there are subclassifications and variations on the basic structure. In general, however, HMOs, PPOs, and other managed care structures (e.g., exclusive provider organizations and point-of-service plans) combine mandates for discounts from providers with financial incentives that essentially reward the professional who uses the most efficient and least costly form of diagnosis and treatment.

Managed Care and the Physician-Patient Relationship

The myriad of managed care models impinges on the physician-patient relationship in a variety of ways. There is, however, one common denominator to all of the models, and that is that managed care actively promotes conservative care. This is not intended to impugn a conservative approach to care. Certainly, it is unethical to deliberately withhold needed care. It is also unethical to knowingly provide unnecessary care. Traditional fee-for-service delivery systems are capable of negatively affecting the doctor-patient relationship by inserting a financial conflict of interest. For example, such delivery systems can promote overutilization associated with third-party reimbursement practices and their passing the balance due on to the patient. In response to criticism of overutilization, the physician can easily externalize the cost factor component by maintaining that the test or procedure or length of stay was medically necessary to "maximize diagnostic and therapeutic certainty." As malpractice litigation continues to rise, this becomes an increasingly defensible rationale. Further, patients are less likely to complain about the inconvenience of excessive testing and its questionable benefit and more likely to be comforted by the technology. Put another way, patients are less likely to be concerned about false positive results and the related anxiety of excessive testing than about the possibility of missed diagnoses pursuant to conservative utilization of testing. Hence, the stage is set for an intraindividual conflict to develop among patients: As members of society and health care consumers in the abstract, individuals generally concur with the need for cost containment efforts. As persons in actual need of medical attention, these same individuals want to retain the same options and ready access to utilization of benefits under managed care as they had under traditional fee-for-service arrangements.

As previously stated, ethical aspects of the physician-patient relationship have traditionally focused on the moral responsibilities of individual physicians to individual patients. We believe that the physician's *primary* ethical duty should remain with the individual patient, and, secondarily, to the interests of patients as a group to whom ethical duties are also owed. In our view, the trust that individual personal commitment engenders and the advocacy that this represents forms the foundation of the physician-patient relationship. However, this position is becoming increasingly difficult to actualize. As set forth in the AMA Council on Ethical and Judicial Affairs draft report (American Medical Association 1994), managed care creates at least two conflicting loyalties for the physician: 1) physicians are expected to balance the interests of their patients with the interests of other patients (e.g., prioritizing resource allocation), and 2) managed care can place needs of patients in conflict with the financial interests of their physicians (e.g., the use of bonuses and fee withholds to reward cost-conscious, fiscally conservative behaviors). Both areas are discussed further later on.

Conflicts Among Patients/Resource Allocation Decisions

Managed care can generate conflicts of loyalty for physicians in terms of advocacy priorities for their individual patients as measured against the needs and interests of other patients. Managed care plans often contain allocation guidelines that set forth which service should be provided for a given group of patients who share certain clinical characteristics. The amount of independent physician discretion varies among plan types. Hence, an intraindividual conflict among physicians arises: A "bedside rationing" role is being asked of the physician, which is in direct conflict with the physician's traditional role of advocate for an individual patient in terms of what would best materially benefit that particular patient. That is to say, this type of gate-keeping, managed care role generates a conflict "between the responsibilities of the physician as a primary advocate of the patient and guardian of society's resources" (American Medical Association 1994).

Notwithstanding physicians' obligations to society, it is fundamental that they not lose sight of their ethical mandate to be primarily dedicated to the health needs of their individual patients. The AMA report sets forth suggestions whereby physicians can preserve their role of providing treatment that will materially benefit their patients while not withholding treatment to preserve the plan's resources. One means is for physicians to "contribute their expertise in the development of [clinical] guidelines" and to "advocate for the consideration of differences among patients" (American Medical Association 1994). We concur with this. Clinical practice guidelines are becoming increasingly popular. Essentially, they set forth consistent approaches to treatment of specific diseases. They have proven to be effective cost containment efforts by expediting diagnostic evaluations and consequently the pace of treatment. However, it is imperative that the concern over the utilization of such guidelines not be actualized (i.e., the reduction of the practice of clinical medicine to a "cookbook" methodology). This is critical in all specialty areas and particularly so in psychiatry, where individual differences in factors related to the development or expression of psychiatric symptomatology may significantly impact on the type and timing of therapeutic interventions.

Another means recommended by the AMA through which physicians may preserve their role in relation to individual patients is to continue to uphold their duty to "advocate for the individual's right to treatment in any case where material benefit to a particular patient would result" (American Medical Association 1994), notwithstanding the recommendations or prohibitions of the managed care plan. In the authors' opinion, this can be accomplished in fact and is not merely an academically idealistic proposal. To facilitate such an outcome, the AMA has proposed legislation that would require managed care organizations to include three physician members on the plan's governing board in addition to a medical board composed entirely of participating physicians (American Medical Association 1994). The physicians would be responsible for periodic review of restrictions on services and other coverage-related matters. Such medical review panels would appropriately insert the professional medical views of physicians in decision making directly associated with the provision of medical care and provide potential support to the individual physician in his or her advocacy role.

The AMA report also recommends that patients play an active part in preserving the role of the physician in relation to individual patients. This would be in the form of patient participation in coverage-related decision making pursuant to plan benefits. Such involvement requires the patients to be adequately informed about proposed and existing coverage provisions of their plans. The importance of patient knowledge and awareness of plan benefits cannot be overemphasized.

In the authors' view, the process of disclosure in general is the sine qua non of preserving the ethical obligation of physicians toward their patients in the era of managed care. This process is more thoroughly discussed in the section on informed consent and managed care.

Conflicts Between Physicians and Patients

The second area of conflicting physician loyalty related to managed care concerns ethical problems associated with financial incentives to limit care. Specifically, physicians are induced to contain cost through the use of such incentives as bonuses and fee withholds that directly affect income. The AMA report notes that such incentives are not per se unethical but can be so used (American Medical Association 1994). An example would be for a primary care physician to wait a longer period of time before ordering additional tests or initiating a referral to a specialist on the basis of anticipated negative personal financial consequences of such actions (American Medical Association 1994). Physicians who may be at particular risk to be challenged in reference to issues of financial conflict and loyalty toward their patients are arguably those who engage in any combination of treatment models in which physicians are simultaneously treating both fee-for-service and managed care plan clients. These "double agent" physicians may be perceived as adjusting the standard of care to the benefit plan for personal financial reasons to the medical detriment of the patient. Notwithstanding the existence of a legitimate medical rationale for differential treatment among patients with similar presenting symptoms and disorders, to the extent that there is an appearance that the provisions of a benefit plan are driving the physician's approach to treatment (e.g., its type and duration), such differential treatment by the same physician becomes less defensible. This is an important issue because it potentially affects many physicians. Unless a single payer model of health reform is instituted, which is unlikely at this time, the majority of physicians' practices will probably contain, at least for a period of time, a mix of managed care and traditional indemnity patients.

Ethicist E. Haavi Morreim has developed an interesting and compelling approach to addressing conflicts between physicians and patients (Morreim 1989). She begins with the premise that the distribution of medical resources is an uneven one that has led to a differential of medical and monetary resource availability across socioeconomic strata. This she terms "stratified scarcity" (Morreim 1989). As a consequence of stratified scarcity and the resulting managed care responses to it, physicians can no longer conform to a traditional application of the standard of care, which is that physicians are required to deliver to all of their patients "a roughly equal minimum quality of care" (Morreim 1989). Because physicians can no longer exert the same degree of control over fiscal and medical resources, the exertion of such equality is no longer possible. In response, Dr. Morreim proposes a major reorganization of the concept of the standard of care, in which the standard is divided into two separate but interrelated elements: 1) the "standard of medical expertise" (SME), which is the traditional standard of professional knowledge and expertise owed to patients by their physicians and 2) the "standard of resource use" (SRU), which addresses medical judgments in conjunction with third parties' economic determinations about what resources can be afforded (Morreim 1989).

With regard to the SME, under a divided standard of care, physicians would be held, as before, to possess the same level of medical expertise as other members of the field according to a national standard of "accepted practice" (Morreim 1989). Under the bifurcated standard, however, before proceeding solely on the basis of medical necessity, the physician must actively consider the extent of financial resources available to be spent on the patient's health care needs. This is the standard of resource use (SRU), and it is at this juncture factored into the medical decision-making analysis. Dr. Morreim correctly points out that to make a medical decision is to make a spending decision and that consequently it is appropriate for physicians to take resource availability into account (Morreim 1989). By her analogy, if physicians are precluded from imposing unwanted treatment on unconsenting patients, so too should they be prevented from distributing others' money and property without consent (Morreim 1989).

The physician does not lose his or her individual advocacy duties of care under the SRU. Indeed, Morreim holds that it is "incumbent upon physicians to work with third-party payers to ensure that economic protocols guiding resource utilization are medically appropriate" (Morreim 1989). Specifically, the SRU requires that a part of the physician's duty to an individual patient be an advisory component in terms of reviewing the various intervention options available, including those that may not be covered under the terms of the patient's benefit plan. As Morreim observes, the physician's SME and SRU obligations directly overlap at this juncture, insofar as the patient is being assisted in making decisions in light of both relevant medical facts and economic reality (Morreim 1989).

Professor Morreim does not leave the physician-patient relationship standing alone in terms of ethical duties and responsibilities under the SRU. She attaches such obligations to third-party payers as well, with the nexus being the contractual terms of the agreement with the patient. In her model, managed care plan providers would have a duty to the patient to negotiate honestly and carry out contractual commitments in good faith. Further, ambiguities in the plans should be settled in favor of the subscriber's "reasonable expectations" of coverage. Whereas patients usually do not and cannot negotiate the terms of their own health resource contracts, she notes that they nonetheless have viable remedies through which to seek enforcement of duties owed. One such method is to negotiate in groups for interpretations of any changes in benefit provisions. In this regard, Morreim points out the readiness of courts to honor the "reasonable expectations" of insurance subscribers (Morreim 1989). By actively factoring the contractual relationship between the patient and third party into the SRU and thus acknowledging the reality of stratified scarcity, Morreim argues that the physician may be morally obliged to provide the best health care possible but should not be held legally accountable (in a standard of care analysis) for failure to deliver resources for which no one is willing to pay, a situation entirely outside of the physician's control (Morreim 1989). The issue of physician accountability in the face of limited resources is discussed in the section on informed consent as it relates to disclosure responsibilities, appeal responsibilities, and continuation of treatment responsibilities.

Others have emphasized the moral components of managed care plans. Pellegrino and Thomasma express the opinion that to the extent that the managed care plan assumes 1) a duty to a level of skill or competence; 2) a duty to make that skill level maximally available to the patient; and 3) a duty to act as the patient's advocate, the plan is functioning as a fiduciary or "moral agent" in health care, thus sharing the obligation of the traditional moral agent, the physician (Pellegrino and Thomasma 1981).

However, as Morreim points out, there are legal implications based in tort law associated with holding managed care provider plans accountable to patients under the medical profession's standard of care. For example, if managed care plans were held to this standard of care, such an attribution could result in corporate practice of medicine actions. In addition, such a standard would likely require a specified minimum benefit plan, which has been specifically rejected by the United States Supreme Court as applicable to the government (Alexander v Choate 1985). Finally, to the extent that a medical standard would require payers to provide a uniform level of access to health care resources, the result could place unreasonable economic burdens on the plans and ultimately on subscribers (Morreim 1989). Such a result would defeat a primary purpose of managed care: cost containment.

Clearly, the physician conflict issue is a complex one that cannot be easily or quickly resolved. Before leaving this area, one area of physician-patient conflict particularly relevant to psychiatry should be noted. This concerns the implicit pressure to expand concepts and definitions of mental illness in response to economic pressure to diagnose more mental illness in order to fill inpatient beds (Morreim 1990). Further, the patient may even be the source of pressure to hospitalize when such is not clinically indicated, if inpatient care offers a better benefit option than an outpatient forum. Psychiatrists are thus placed in ethical conflict over addressing the patient's medical welfare in ways appropriate to the practice of their profession versus responding to the patient's economic concerns by "gaming the system" (Morreim 1991).

In the authors' views, for the physician-patient relationship to remain viable, it is imperative that physicians first establish and then not compromise a sense of trust with their individual patients. The AMA report advises several means through which physicians may preserve their role and eliminate inappropriate conflicts based on financial factors. One way is to devise incentives that are quality and not quantity based (i.e., to reinforce and reward "appropriate" professional behavior, which would result in punishing "inappropriate" services [American Medical Association 1994]). Examples of quality measures are objective outcomes data (e.g., mortality and morbidity); extent of adherence to practice guidelines or other approved standards of care; patient satisfaction; and peer review (American Medical Association 1994).

Managed Care and Informed Consent

As previously set forth, standards of informed consent include the professional or "reasonable physician" standard, the "materiality" or "patient-centered" standard and, in some jurisdictions, a hybrid form involving both. Pursuant to the "new ethics" embodied by health care reform requirements, the authors recommend that the standard applied in managed care circumstances be a hybrid form. In our view, utilizing a professional-only standard does not adequately address the physician-patient conflict potential. Utilization of the "reasonable physician" standard alone has the potential to reflect the best interests of the physician at the expense of the patient's interests. However, utilization of a professional standard as a component of a broader patient-inclusive standard allows for the retention of a certain amount of physician beneficence, which the author views as desirable in a managed care setting. As suggested by Professor Susan Wolf, "Fully informing the patient of the potentially beneficial treatment options and the pros and cons of each allows the patient to form a therapeutic alliance with the physician and to make informed choices" (Wolf 1994). A patient-centered standard imposes a duty to disclose and discuss features and options of the plan that a reasonable patient would want to know. Incorporating both standards sets forth a higher threshold of informed consent, which is desirable at a time of transition in health care where choice is at a minimum.

Wolf further notes the importance of including economic and other barriers a patient may encounter in obtaining a particular treatment as part of the disclosure process (Wolf 1994). This should include *all* potentially beneficial treatments, regardless of whether they are covered by the patient's plan. This enables the patient to challenge or appeal the provisions of his or her plan, while providing the patient the maximum amount of information upon which to evaluate available options.

The authors strongly endorse the practice of full disclosure to patients, and that is the inclusion of clinical and nonclinical information (e.g., particulars of benefit information). These particulars, sometimes referred to as "fiscal informed consent," are essential for the physician to fully discharge the duty to provide informed consent. To be specific, at the outset of therapy, clinicians should discuss with a new patient the potential effects of managed care on the course of treatment, including the possibility that payment for treatment might be terminated before either the patient or the therapist believes that the goals of treatment have been realized. As Appelbaum points out, "Patients who are about to embark on therapy involving painful self-disclosure and the activation of disturbing affects, might well find such information important to proceed" (Applebaum 1993).

If subsequent denial of benefits should occur, the clinician will need to revisit the issue and review available options with the patient. Such options include the assumption of a self-pay arrangement or transferring to an alternate source of care. By reviewing the components of the patient's plan at the outset of treatment and discussing the issue as needed in the course of treatment, the clinician is actively addressing resource utilization responsibilities. It is important to note, Appelbaum points out, that the duty to disclose in a managed care context is not one in which the courts have ruled on, and thus its status is unclear (Appelbaum 1993).

Courts have suggested, however, that clinicians have an affirmative duty to appeal adverse managed care treatment decisions. In *Wickline v. State,* one of the leading managed care cases, the California Court of Appeals stated, "[T]he physician who complies without protest with the limitations imposed by a third party payer, when his medical judgment dictates otherwise, cannot avoid his ultimate responsibility for the patient's care" (Wickline v State 1986). We concur with a recommendation for physician advocacy in the face of economically driven decisions that may threaten to compromise patient care, even though such action raises additional questions (e.g., how far should the advocacy extend, and how many levels of appeals should be pursued?).

In addition to having a duty to appeal adverse decisions, physicians have been found to have a duty to continue treatment following managed care denial of benefit determinations. In *Varol v. Blue Cross and Blue Shield of Michigan,* the court stated, "Whether or not the proposed treatment is approved, the physician retains the right and indeed the ethical and legal obligation to provide appropriate treatment to the patient" (Vard v Blue Cross and Blue Shield of Michigan 1989). Appelbaum points out that the imposition of a duty to continue treatment is not an absolute one and is not sustainable as a matter of public policy (Appelbaum 1993). We concur with this, notwithstanding the physician's duties, 1) not to abandon a patient, 2) to advocate on the patient's behalf, and 3) to discuss and disclose the economic consequences of their treatment decisions (Morreim 1989). This position is a rational and defensible one in our view and in accordance with the bifurcated standard of care model, in which the physician is not expected to be indefinitely responsible for circumstances such as the particulars of a patient's benefit plan over which he or she has virtually no control (Morreim 1989).

Two final points need to be made about the importance of disclosure. First, disclosure is a major focus of the Patient Protection Act, federal legislation that addresses patient access to care proposed by the AMA in 1994 (Patient Protection Act of 1994). Under its terms, the Secretary of Health and Human Services (HHS) would develop federal standards for the certification of managed care plans. In order to be certified, plans would have to provide information to prospective enrollees about the terms and conditions of the plan in order to enable enrollees to make informed decisions about accepting a certain system of health care delivery. The act further requires that where the plan is described orally to enrollees, easily understood, truthful, and objective terms must be used. The specific provisions for patient protection under the act include requirements that information be provided on the following:

1. Coverage provisions, benefits, and any exclusions by category of service, provider, or physician, and, where applicable, by specific service
2. Any and all prior authorization or other review requirements including preauthorization review, concurrent review, postservice review, postpayment review, and any procedures that may cause the patient to be denied coverage for or not be provided a particular service
3. Financial arrangements or contractual provisions with hospitals, review companies, physicians, or any other provider of health care services that would limit the services offered, restrict referral or treatment options, or negatively affect the physician's fiduciary responsibility to his or her patients, including but not limited to financial incentives not to provide medical or other services
4. Explanation of how plan limitations impact enrollees, including information on enrollee financial responsibility for payment for coinsurance or other noncovered or out-of-plan services
5. Loss ratios
6. Enrollee satisfaction statistics

Finally, the importance of disclosure to the AMA is illustrated in its draft Report of the Council of Ethical and Judicial Affairs, in which the AMA recommends that disclosure pursuant to physician financial incentives to limit care be fully disclosed to patients by plan administrators upon enrollment and at least annually thereafter (American Medical Association 1994).

Managed Care and Confidentiality

A major component of health reform proposals includes the need to reduce the costs of administering the medical record-keeping system (Alpert 1994). As a means to achieve savings, most reform proposals rely on computer technology to both maintain medical record information and to expeditiously transfer such information to those who "need to know" (Alpert 1994). As previously noted, the confidentiality requirements of mental health-related information are greater than those of general medical information. The computerization of mental health records potentially compromises providers' ability to adequately protect this sensitive information. The reason to adopt a more efficient means of record keeping (i.e., more efficient than the cumbersome nature and related expense of the traditional paper method) actually offers a form of protection against breaches of confidentiality. The electronic medium potentially allows for relatively easy unauthorized access, both intentionally and inadvertently (Alpert 1994). The possible consequences of such breaches in psychiatry are significant. First, and most importantly, a patient's fundamental need for trust in his or her psychiatrist as a precondition to discussing extremely personal and sensitive medical information without fear of others having access to such information is jeopardized (Alpert 1994). As one physician stated, "Our once-sacred relationship is engaged to marry the technology of the information age" (Alpert 1994). Second, if patients, in conjunction with their psychiatrists, cannot adequately control the access and distribution of their mental health records, this could actively deter patients from seeking psychiatric assistance at all or prolong such consultation. This result is certainly not in the patient's best interest from a medical/psychiatric perspective; nor is it in the interest of the psychiatrist from a standard of care perspective; nor is it in the managed care plan's interests from either a cost-saving or a public relations perspective.

The inability of psychiatrists and patients to adequately control access to medical record information could also result in patients' being less than forthcoming with their psychiatrist. This would clearly serve to undercut a potentially major benefit of the computerization of medical records (i.e., to efficiently and expeditiously make available to other physicians and providers, who are actively or emergently engaged in the treatment of the patient, a thorough and up-to-date account of the patient's medical history and present treatment). The authors maintain, therefore, that it is in the interest of all three parties to ensure that confidentiality issues are adequately addressed before the "information superhighway" becomes an unalterable reality.

As a means by which a balance between an individual's legitimate need for privacy can be weighed against the need for personal identifying medical information to be communicated to the medical community, insurance company, or managed care organization, some have proposed that federal legislation addressing patient privacy and medical information practices be enacted. This is reasonable in view of the fact that "the current patchwork of state laws, court decisions, and limited federal regulations cannot assure a legally guaranteed set of rights that will place the individual on a much more level playing field with those having access to his or her medical information" (Alpert 1994).

Alpert (1994) proposes one of the most comprehensive plans for federal privacy legislation. It is based on the Privacy Protection Study Commission of 1977, created after the passage of the Privacy Act, and requires that such federal legislation should:

1. clearly define the rights patients have with respect to their own medical information;
2. define what constitutes legitimate access to and use of personal health and medical information, as well as specifying prohibited uses;
3. provide oversight and enforcement mechanisms to ensure compliance;
4. establish civil and criminal penalties for prohibited activities to enable patients to collect damages;
5. establish medical record retention schedules for each class of information recipient (i.e., physicians, hospitals, insurers, etc.);
6. require that patients be notified of the use to which information in health and medical records is put and how patients may obtain their medical records;
7. require extensive audit trails accessible to patients upon request, to track all disclosures and requests for disclosure of personal medical information, including the reasons for which the information was requested;
8. apply to all health care providers;
9. establish a totally unique patient identification scheme that prohibits all other uses not directly related to providing medical care;
10. strictly limit employers' ability to see individual employees' medical/health records and use them to make employment-related decisions;

11. prohibit "pretext interviews," where an insurer or employer conducts an investigation into a patient's medical history under false pretenses in order to gain access to health records;
12. prohibit the marketing of personal health-medical data; and
13. give patients the prerogative to limit the authorization for the use and disclosure of their medical record information (to include specific references to the records subject to authorization, the parties allowed access, an expiration date for the authorization, and a right to revoke that authorization).

The authors recommend that the enactment of federal legislation be advocated by patients, physicians, and managed care organizations alike. Realistically, however, even if privacy legislation is passed, significant compromises in the inclusive criteria suggested by Alpert may need to occur as a condition of passage. In the interim, physicians should make every effort to fulfill their professional duty of confidentiality toward their patients pursuant to federal and state privacy laws, physician or psychotherapist-client privilege statutes, and the common law.

As previously indicated, a generally recognized exception to the requirement of patient consent for the release of confidential information is third-party payers for reimbursement purposes. Generally, the information to which this exception applies refers to "staff names, dates, types and costs of therapies or services and a short description of the general purposes of each treatment session or service" (Pennsylvania Mental Health Procedures Act 1993). With its need for much more specific and detailed information in order to conduct a thorough review of the case in terms of whether the diagnosis and proposed treatment warrant reimbursement, managed care extends this exception beyond its limited parameters and, according to some, is bringing about the erosion of the confidentiality privilege. To minimize or prevent such a result, the authors support Appelbaum's "rule of austerity" (i.e., providing the minimum necessary data to answer the question posed by the third party [Appelbaum 1991]). In addition, to the extent possible, the patient should not only be informed about the need to advance certain clinical information to a representative from his or her benefit plan but should be offered the opportunity to review such information in collaboration with the physician. The clinical status of the patient and/or logistical time factors may preclude this process. Patients need to be made aware of what the information requirements are pursuant to their plans and the scope of their plan's definition of "for reimbursement purposes." Managed care organizations should be precluded from re-release of confidential information without the patient's consent and should be held accountable for deliberate or inadvertent breaches under a violation of contract theory, applying Morreim's contract theory of patient-owed duties by managed care organizations.

Conclusion

As a result of health care reform initiatives in general and managed care plan agreements in particular, the physician-patient relationship is undergoing significant changes. Physicians are functioning in roles as providers of services, managed care reviewers, managers or owners of managed care companies, network developers, competitors, and subspecialists, to name a few of their many roles. Accordingly, the integrity of the traditional physician-patient relationship is being threatened. Further, privacy and confidentiality are compromised by plan administrators' needs for extensive clinical information as a precondition of payment at all points of treatment. Trust, an essential factor in the development of a therapeutic alliance, which in psychiatry is especially instrumental to the healing process, is more difficult both to establish and to maintain. Moreover, the physician's duty to provide informed consent as traditionally developed to relate to clinical matters needs to be broadened in scope in the face of the economic realities attendant to managed care plan benefit terms. In this chapter we have argued that the fundamental duty of physicians has been and should remain one of advocacy on behalf of the individual patient's best interest. Moral obligations toward patients should not be viewed in terms of an "either-or" beneficent or self-determination perspective but needs to contain aspects of each. By restoring aspects of beneficence to the physician-patient relationship, physicians will be able to respond affirmatively to the challenges of managed care and more actively address their professional ethical duties toward patients to avoid harm and injustice. Through such affirmative actions, patient advocacy may prevail over indifference.

References

Alexander v Choate, 105 US 712 (1985)
Alpert S: Smart cards, smarter policy—medical records, privacy, and healthcare reform. Hastings Cent Rep 23:13, 1994
American Medical Association. Principles of Medical Ethics, Current Opinions of the Judicial Council. American Medical Association, Chicago, IL, 1984
American Medical Association. Ethical issues in managed care, in Report on the Council of Ethical and Judicial Affairs (CEJA), 13-A-94. American Medical Association, 1994
Appelbaum PS: Legal liability and managed care. Am Psychol 48:251, 1993
Appelbaum PS, Gutheil TG: Clinical Handbook of Psychiatry and the Law. Baltimore, MD, Williams & Wilkins, 1991
Appelbaum PS, Lidz CW, Meisel A: Informed Consent—Legal Theory and Clinical Practice. New York, Oxford University Press, 1987
Beauchamp TL, McCullough LB: Medical Ethics—The Moral Responsibilities of Physicians. Englewood Cliffs, NJ, Prentice-Hall, 1984
Canterbury v Spence, 464 DC 772 (1972)
Congressional Budget Office (CBO) Staff Memorandum: The Effects of Managed Care on Use and Costs of Health Services. Washington, DC, Congressional Budget Office, June 1992
Feldman JL, Fitzpatrick RJ (eds): Managed Mental Health Care—Administrative and Clinical Issues. Washington, DC, American Psychiatric Press, 1992
Klerman GL, Weissman MM, Appelbaum, et al. (eds): Social, Epidemiologic, and Legal Psychiatry, Philadelphia, PA, JB Lippincott, 1986
Morreim EH: Stratified scarcity: redefining the standard of care. Law Med Health Care 17:356–367, 1989
Morreim EH: The new economics of medicine: special changes to psychiatry. J Med Philos 15:98, 1990
Morreim EH: Economic disclosure and economic advocacy—new duties in the medical standard of care. J Leg Med 12:275–329, 1991a
Morreim EH: Gaming the system. Arch Intern Med 151:443, 1991b

Natansan v Kline, 350 KS 1093, 1960
Pellegrino ED, Thomasma DC: A Philosophical Basis of Medical Practice. New York, Oxford University Press, 1981
Pennsylvania Mental Health Procedures Act: 55 Pa. Code §5100.32(a)(2), 1993
Salgo v Leland Stanford Junior University Board of Trustees, 317 CA 170, 181 (1957)
U.S. House of Representatives: Patient Protection Act of 1994. 103d Cong., 1st sess., H.R. 4527, 1994 Vard v Blue Cross and Blue Shield of Michigan, 708 F. Supp. 826 (E.D. Mich. 1989)
Webb WL: Ethical psychiatric practice in a new economic climate. Psychiatric Annals 19:443–447, 1989
Wickline v State, 228 CA 661 (1986)
Wolf SM: Health care reform and the future of physician ethics. Hastings Cent Rep 24:35, 1994

CHAPTER TEN

New Financial Incentives and Disincentives in Psychiatry

Jeremy A. Lazarus, M.D.

> The profit motive without moral guidance is blind; moral inspiration without financial backing is bankrupt.
>
> —H. Tristram Engelhardt Jr., Ph.D., M.D., and Michael A. Rie, M.D.

Before the onset of third-party reimbursement for medical care, payment for medical services was based on a contractual relationship between doctor and patient. Patients relied on physicians to use their best judgment and beneficence to treat them—following a tradition of a covenant between doctor and patient to do no harm and always act in the best interest of the patient. In return, the patient compensated the physician directly with some form of payment.

As medical care has become more expensive in the last 50 years, third-party reimbursement has emerged as the most likely method of payment for medical services. For example, Blue Cross/Blue Shield plans entered the scene in the thirties and forties, albeit with AMA opposition. Although patients have assumed less and less direct responsibility for payment for services, they continue to assume that the physician has the same covenant relationship with them (Mechanic et al. 1990).

Physicians have always generated income predominantly by direct patient payment and insurance reimbursement, but over the last century some physicians have increased their income in ways that indicate inherent conflicts of interest. In his book *Medicine, Money, and Morals* (1993), Rodwin has compiled descriptions of these methods; here are the most common:

1. Receiving kickbacks for referrals
2. Referring patients to medical facilities in which the doctors themselves invest (physician self-referral)
3. Dispensing drugs, selling medical products, and performing ancillary medical services
4. Selling medical practices to hospitals
5. Accepting payments made by hospitals to recruit and bond physicians
6. Accepting gifts from medical suppliers

The AMA has addressed these conflict-of-interest situations with written guidelines and codes, although slowly. The medical profession has resisted regulation, relying instead on physicians' morals to prevail. Nevertheless, according to Rodwin, various forms of fee-splitting were common up until the fifties. As incidents of medical, including psychiatric, fraud became more publicized in the late eighties, physicians started to become primary targets for blame. Many of the scandals involved physicians who engineered highly profitable, scientifically corrupt schemes. The purpose of this chapter is not to focus on such clearly fraudulent behavior but to explore the new financial incentives and disincentives that affect psychiatric practice. It is to elucidate differences in psychiatric practice financially and to determine why it is important to examine incentives and suggestions for an approach that will limit physicians' conflicts of interest and motivate improved care.

The Spectrum of Financial Incentives and Disincentives in Medicine

The Health Maintenance Act of 1973 specifically required health maintenance organizations (HMOs) to use physician incentives as a means of reducing medical costs. However, the new financial incentives and disincentives in medicine stem from managed care, or managed competition, the primary purpose of which is to constrain the rising costs of health care. Managed care companies provide physicians with financial incentives and disincentives as a way to cut costs. Numerous incentives are available to primary care physicians and a more limited number to specialists. Hillman lists various incentives:

- *Capitation:* A method of payment by which the physician receives a periodic fee for each enrollee to cover all care required.
- *Salary:* A method of payment by which the physician is remunerated at a constant rate on a regular basis.
- *Withhold:* A percentage of the physician's payment is retained against a potential deficit in the referral funds.
- *Bonus:* The sharing of a surplus in the referral funds with the physician.
- *Bonus based on productivity:* An extra payment to the physician that is based in part on a measure of productivity.
- *Risk beyond withhold (specialist fund):* A financial risk assumed by the physician who is subject to withholding, in the event of a deficit in the specialist referral fund over and above the loss of withheld funds; or a financial risk assumed by the physician who is subject to withholding, in the event of a deficit in the hospital referral fund over and above the loss of withheld funds.
- *Individual risk:* A financial risk assumed by the physician in the event of a deficit in the referral fund, calculated on the basis of individual performance.
- *Ancillary risk:* A financial risk assumed by the physician when payment for outpatient tests is made out of funds otherwise designated for payment to the physician.
- *Specialist risk:* A financial risk assumed by specialists in order to share in the risk-bonus structure.

Additional incentives not included by Hillman include the following:

- Increased patient volume guaranteed with discounted fees
- Employment promotion based on cost savings or other performance measures
- Profit-sharing in the stock of the company
- Equity shares of the company worked for or with
- Retainers, a fixed amount of income for a fixed number of patients referred
- Case rate, a fixed amount of income for a specific case, based on diagnosis or treatment setting (e.g., outpatient or inpatient)

Disincentives include the following:

- Limits on admitting privileges
- Removal from panels of physician providers
- Financial sanctions
- Termination of employment
- Decreased reimbursement

It is in the best financial interest of third-party owners of health plans to spend as little as possible on medical services without dissatisfying their customers (Relman 1991). Incentives they impose on their physicians can further this goal. If these incentives cause physicians to neglect their primary role of advocate for their patients, an ethical dilemma results (Thompson 1993). These incentives may then force physicians to trade in their social contracts for business contracts (Relman and Reinhardt 1986).

One other common financial incentive is a form of gatekeeping in which a primary care physician controls access to specialists and services and is "rewarded" with moneys not spent. Pellagrino, a foremost medical ethicist, describes three forms of gatekeeping (Pellagrino 1986):

> The first is the traditional, or *de facto* function, which imposes a responsibility to practice rational medicine, i.e., to use only those diagnostic and therapeutic modalities beneficial and effective for the patient. The proper exercise of traditional gatekeeping is not only morally imperative but economically sound.
>
> The second form of gatekeeping is the negative gatekeeping role, usually within some form of prepayment system in which the physician strives to limit the use of health care services. This role is morally dubious because it generates a conflict between the responsibilities of the physician as a primary advocate of the patient and as guardian of society's resources. Under certain carefully defined conditions of economic necessity and moral monitoring, a negative gatekeeping role might be morally justifiable.
>
> The third form of gatekeeping is positive gatekeeping in which the physician encourages the use of health care facilities and services for personal or corporate profit. This is an indefensible form of gatekeeping. No moral justification can be mustered in its favor.

Interestingly, there is no firm evidence that negative gatekeeping affects cost savings (Azevedo 1994).

To discourage physicians from limiting services, the managed care industry has taken steps to predict and minimize the financial risk of patients (Kralewski 1994). One way to lower financial risk that could materialize from particularly risky patients would be to replace patient prepayment with negotiated fee-for-service payment with a high holdback (up to 20%) distributed at year's end. The money withheld would be distributed based on a formula comparing the plan's physicians in this arrangement to one another. Those who generated the most profit would receive the largest distributions. This approach is fraught with ethical dilemmas (e.g., some physicians not generating the most profits might be more effectively treating their patients but would be penalized because patient outcome is not factored in).

Other approaches are based on capitation with risk-sharing mechanisms that protect physicians from particularly adverse patient selection. For example, incentives for physicians that are spread over a larger group of patients create less risk for the physician. Nevertheless, the potential to underutilize services for the purpose of financial gain still exists. Prearranged utilization targets tied to physician compensation likewise create conflict (Hillman et al. 1989). With the recent debate over health care reform, ethicists have been discussing this conflict of interest (Wolf 1994). The American College of Physicians and the AMA assert that physicians should advocate for their patients even in the face of financial incentives that encourage them not to (American College of Physicians 1992; American Medical Association 1995). Unfortunately, the AMA and APA have not yet determined which financial incentives are acceptable and which are not. Perhaps part of the delay stems from the fact that it is not yet clear whether managed care financial arrangements diminish quality of care and patient outcome (Safran et al. 1994).

Physicians who face financial incentives and disincentives that discourage optimal care have an obligation to rise above the profit motive and serve as advocates for their patients. Nonmedical ethicists and the medical profession have made it clear that physicians have an ethical obligation to help patients obtain all services to which they are legally and economically entitled (American Medical Association 1994;

Morreim 1991). According to Susan Wolf, "[t]he physician should have a presumptive duty to strive to provide treatments that are potentially beneficial and chosen by informed patients or proper surrogates. Categories of 'potentially beneficial treatment' will have to be enumerated. They should at minimum include (1) treatments empirically demonstrated to provide benefit valued by patients (how often the treatment must be provided and with what size benefit would have to be determined); (2) treatments regarded as part of the standard of care for a given condition (a standard that would, of course, change over time with the advent of new information and techniques); and (3) treatments recommended by established clinical practice guidelines."

When health plans limit treatment, physicians should inform patients of all potentially beneficial treatment and of barriers to that treatment (including contract barriers under the particular plan) or refer them to personnel who can explain the plan, and they should determine how to advocate for patients within the organization. For example, treating psychiatrists must advocate for all medically necessary psychotherapy services as they would for any other medical services. And that applies equally to psychiatrist administrators and utilization reviewers (American Medical Association 1993). Although other mental health professionals can also provide psychotherapy services in managed care settings, it is crucial that psychiatrists retain their psychotherapeutic skills and not be excluded from providing these services. These parties could have a hard time fulfilling their ethical obligation as patient advocates in the face of financial incentives and disincentives that motivate them not to.

The Spectrum of Incentives and Disincentives in Psychiatry

The managed care and behavioral health care industries have created psychiatric "carve outs," due not only to financial motives but at least in part to stigma and inaccurate information regarding psychiatric treatment. Some of these carve-out companies claim that, without their participation in certain prepaid health care systems, treatment for mental illness would be even more compromised. Others raise concerns about overall responsibility in these systems (Lazarus 1994).

Decreased reimbursement to psychiatrists after a fixed number of sessions provides a strong disincentive to psychiatrists to continue beyond that fixed number and creates a significant conflict of interest. Capitation arrangements for psychiatric services have become commonplace in some areas of the country. Under capitation, psychiatric groups, psychiatric hospitals, behavioral health care companies, and other types of organized systems of delivery contract for mental health and substance abuse treatment. Capitation rates vary dramatically and, if inadequate, can have a profound effect on quality and access to treatment.

Some systems provide bonuses or commissions to utilization reviewers for decreasing the number of services provided. Although the bonus may be derived from utilization or medical necessity criteria, it may put pressure on the reviewer to deny services when there is some ambiguity in the criteria or their application. When the bonus is truly tied to use of professionally developed criteria, it may not conflict with the physician's primary role as patient advocate. Yet there are deep concerns that these "market values" are having a deleterious effect on the practice of medicine (Relman 1992).

Some organized psychiatric systems, such as the Harvard Community Health Plan, have applied justice principles in their health care delivery, whereby the most seriously ill benefit the most. In this model, patients with the most severe psychiatric illnesses pay lower copayments than those patients with less severe psychiatric illnesses. Such a system may still provide psychiatrists with incentives to be cost efficient and may be tied to quality parameters.

These factors, among others, have had a dramatic impact on the practice of psychiatry. Combined with incentives and disincentives for managed health care as a whole, they have resulted in large decreases in the length of hospital stays, failure to fund longer-term psychotherapies (and approval in many plans of only the briefest therapy), inclusion of lower-cost providers (especially for psychotherapy services), and exclusion, or limitation on numbers, of psychiatrists from provider panels.

Whereas scientific research is lacking, reaction from within the profession is extensive. The impact of the changes in economics and their influence on ethics in psychiatric care have been described (Lazarus and Sharfstein 1994). Several APA publications have covered ethical issues related to managed care (American Psychiatric Association

Ethics Newsletter 1988, 1992), as have the APA-sponsored conferences on ethics in managed care in 1991 and 1994.

The APA published conflict-of-interest guidelines (American Psychiatric Association Ethics Newsletter 1989) but otherwise has not commented exhaustively on various forms of physician incentives and disincentives. Perhaps more thorough codes and guidelines on managed care in psychiatric settings will be written and enacted when researchers conduct adequately controlled studies across treatment settings, with reasonable control of variables, to determine whether one form of psychiatric service delivery is of better quality than others. Perhaps these or other studies can also determine whether one form of psychiatric service delivery is truly more cost efficient than others when looking at all appropriate variables. Sharfstein recommends a prospective, double-blind follow-up method to evaluate the impact on patients of hospital stays shortened by economic constraints (Sharfstein 1991).

Discussion

The new financial incentives and disincentives threaten to compromise the ethics of psychiatrists and the quality of care they provide. Is there a practical solution that will reduce conflict of interest and improve patient care?

Many organizations provide seminars to help physicians understand and negotiate for capitated contracts. In an article entitled "Breaking the Capitation Bronco" (American Medical Association News 1994), the AMA stated that physicians are content and "making more money" through capitated contracts. The article also presented information on "keys to successful capitation." Omitted from these informative seminars and articles are the ethical dilemmas still confronted in capitated contracts. Although there are attempts to minimize these conflicts, the ethical dimensions of capitation are left out of the discussion. At a minimum, physicians in capitated systems should receive ethics training.

Journal of the American Medical Association editor George Lundberg, proposes "economic informed consent." He states: "In a nonemergency situation, all providers should inform the mentally competent adult patient or guardian of the cost of all professional services, medications, tests, procedures, hospitalization, or whatever and obtain the patient's permission prior to providing the service, no matter who is paying the bill. The purpose of this effort is to share the burden of responsibility for expending resources, to cease rendering futile care, and to curtail sharply inappropriate care or 'medicine at the margins' by exercising prospective interactive responsible physician and patient autonomy." Although ethically sound, this approach puts the burden of disclosure solely on the physician (a time-intensive process) and does not address the ethical dilemmas that might discourage informing the patient of all options.

Another possible solution to the ethical dilemmas is to accept them as part of the changing health care system. Engelhardt and Rie state: "For-profit health care corporations are one of the many expressions of human freedom and as such have a presumptive claim to toleration. . . . [F]or-profit corporations have good reason to defend the interests of patients and the ethical integrity of medicine insofar as doing so will attract patronage." They go on: "Everyone who increases the amount of wealth and services, all else remaining equal, indirectly benefits all. Therefore, be good to people and make money. The allure of profits induces people to invest capital. In the absence of the profit motive (or disinterested altruism), capital can be acquired only by coercion." This statement helps to differentiate business ethics from medical ethics. Although their argument is a sound one in general for tolerance and cautious acceptance of the for-profit motive, they do not clearly address the financial pressures passed on to the physician.

The most extensive discussion of financial incentives and disincentives is in Rodwin's *Medicine, Money, and Morals* (Rodwin 1993). He suggests that one approach to conflicted financial incentives and disincentives is to reduce them by paying physicians by salary or by capitation, which he sees as more neutral in terms of neither over- nor underutilizing. He also proposes limiting inappropriate services by providing incentives for appropriate use and imposing fines for inappropriate use: "[T]he incentive would be linked to the correctness of clinical decisions, not general volume targets."

Rodwin's most persuasive suggestion is that doctors should be required by law to answer to patients in a strictly fiduciary capacity, thereby eliminating financial conflicts of interest. He states: "Herein lies the irony: law and rules are sometimes needed to promote an ethos that is deeper, stronger, and more important than the rules themselves. If physicians were required to act solely in the best interest of their patients, they would have to leave to society means of allocating health care resources, if necessary." Although this is one possible solution, its implementation may be mired in regulation, physician oversight of an intrusive nature, and increased administrative costs. All of these would engender significant resistance in the physician population.

Even an outspoken critic of market values in medicine has seen some wisdom in capitated systems. Relman states: "In my opinion, a greater reliance on group practice and more emphasis on medical insurance that prepays providers at a fixed annual rate offer the best chance of solving the economic problems of health care, because these arrangements put physicians in the most favorable position to act as prudent advocates for their patients, rather than as entrepreneurial vendors of services" (Relman 1992). Although Relman may be correct, group practices and capitation in and of themselves would not likely solve the economic problems of health care without other massive adjustments in societal values and probable allocation of resources.

Some physicians have suggested incentives at least partially based on quality (Baker and Brink 1994). They propose evaluation of a sample of patients against the best medical practices for each condition. The problem is that, although physicians would get one score based on quality, their score for efficiency would be based solely on financial impact. The balancing of these two possible incentives deserves more careful thought and study.

Some health plans use "report cards" based on utilization patterns and patient satisfaction. They award bonuses based on "grades" (Azevedo 1994).

Suggested Solutions

I propose a series of approaches to incentives and disincentives that would 1) assist clinicians, as well as those in administrative positions, in maintaining a position of patient advocacy, 2) provide incentives to physicians based primarily on quality of treatment rather than cost containment, and 3) place the ethical dilemmas brought about by increasing health care costs where they belong—with the American public. These approaches apply to psychiatric and behavioral health care systems *and* to health care systems in general.

In the first approach, patients would be offered two basic systems of care: one in which physicians maintain a position of advocacy for patients at all times, regardless of cost, and a second in which physicians advocate for patients within the confines of cost-containment policies (when a group of patients contracts for a system based on just distribution of health care dollars within that system). This could be based on an equality of fair opportunity model described by Daniels (Daniels 1985). This model has also been described in mental health practice (Sabin and Daniels 1994). In this model, patients would receive enough treatment to get them to an opportunity level in their daily life that they would be unable to achieve without such treatment. Alternatively, it could be based on an Oregon allocation-type system based on utilitarian and justice principles in which the health care providers and the consumers together decide on the priorities of covered health care services. Equally acceptable might be other similar innovative systems that use informed consent (the insured group is informed of the ways in which their doctors may consider other factors relating to provision of services, in addition to what is in the patient's best interest). Such a system would have to provide this information to enrollees in understandable language and with full disclosure. In such systems, physicians in administrative and reviewing positions would be held to the same standard of advocacy as clinicians because decision making would clearly be made on justice principles.

But it would be idealistic to expect that all physicians would advocate for patients properly. Rodwin's suggestion to place fiduciary responsibility within the realm of law needs further consideration. If it were developed well, this plan could allow physicians to maintain their ethical covenant with their patients and reduce conflicts of interest to a manageable minimum.

In the second approach, financial incentives would be based primarily (80%–90%) on quality of treatment instead of on cost factors, as most are now. Criteria might include following practice guidelines; achieving scientifically validated, positive clinical outcomes and patient satisfaction; and working collegially in integrated health care systems. Another possibility would be to regulate by statute the caps on physician reimbursement in order to restrict profit or loss under risk-sharing plans. These restrictions would limit payers from providing financial incentives for physicians to change behavior.

In the third approach, physicians would follow specialty-specific guidelines, using medical necessity criteria, and they would be advised to use the most cost-effective treatments that are safe and produce scientifically validated outcomes similar to those of more expensive forms of care. If a system were capitated, it would not be used at the level of the individual physician. There would be risk corridors, through reinsurance, for health care systems to allow for increased income into the capitation pool; if health care providers followed clearly established guidelines and criteria, they would be paid from the system-capitated pool based on how well they followed them. Thus, individual physicians could receive limited bonuses based primarily on quality of treatment.

Finally, utilization review would be done by or under the direction of members of the specialty group; appeals would be presented to objective external third-party specialists. If a system were required to provide more services than projected, its clinicians and administrative physicians would be ethically and/or legally required (because of their fiduciary relationship) to advocate for increased resources.

At this juncture, the public or buyers of a health care system, if there are cost overruns, would need to decide on limiting benefits, eliminating certain services, or providing them at additional cost to the patient. This would place the burden for limitation of services due to economic constraints on the public, where it belongs. Physicians would be involved in those discussions, but ultimately consumers would need to decide. This could lead to an allocation situation such as that recently put into operation in Oregon or to a single-payer system, which has considerable merit. Recent projections of health care costs (Eddy 1994) seem to make it clear that some sort of rationing is inevitable.

The recommendations made would reduce conflicts of interest to a minimum and improve quality of treatment. The approach would require those in positions of influence in organized or managed systems to advocate for patients as a group and to demand the appropriate locus for any allocation of health care resources—to the patients themselves.

Conclusion

This chapter gives a broad overview of financial incentives and disincentives, special problems in psychiatry, and an approach to incentives that would allow physicians to maintain their traditional fiduciary covenant and improve quality of care. It is hoped that psychiatrist clinicians and administrators will be willing to question their motivations and consider replacing current incentives with those proposed in order to improve patient care and retain public trust in the profession.

References

American College of Physician Executives. Perspectives in medical management. Session A-4, 1994
American College of Physicians: Ethics manual, 3rd edition. Ann Intern Med 117:947–960, 1992
American Medical Association: Council on Ethical and Judicial Affairs, Vol IV, No. 1. American Medical Association, Chicago, IL, 1993
American Medical Association: Council on Ethical and Judicial Affairs: Ethical Issues in Managed Care, Report 13-A. American Medical Association, Chicago, IL, 1994
American Medical Association: Ethical issues in managed care. JAMA 273: 330–335, 1995
American Medical News: Breaking the capitation bronco. April 18, 1994, pp 19–20
American Psychiatric Association. Ethics in managed care conference. Baltimore, MD, 1991

American Psychiatric Association. Ethics in managed care conference. Raleigh-Durham, NC, 1994
American Psychiatric Association Ethics Newsletter: New mental health economics and the impact on the ethics of psychiatric practice. Vol IV, No 2, 1988
American Psychiatric Association Ethics Newsletter: Conflicts of interest. 5(2), 1989
American Psychiatric Association Ethics Newsletter: Managed care. Vol VIII, No 1, 1992
Azevedo D: Are we asking too much of gatekeepers? Med Econ, May 22–33, 1994
Baker SR, Brink SD: Why we need quality care nationwide. Bus Health, April 1994, pp 106–107
Daniels N: Just Health Care. Cambridge, MA, Cambridge University Press, 1985
Daniels N: The ideal advocate and limited resources. Theor Med 8:69–80, 1987
Eddy DM: Rationing resources while improving quality: how to get more for less. JAMA 272:817–824, 1994
Engelhardt HT, Rie MA: Morality for the medical-industrial complex. N Engl J Med 319:1086–1089, 1988
General Accounting Office: Outcomes in managed care (report). U.S. General Accounting Office, October 1993
Hillman AL, Pauly MV, Kerstein JJ: How do financial incentives affect physicians' clinical decisions and the financial performance of health maintenance organizations? N Engl J Med 321:86–92, 1989
Jellinek MS, Nurcombe B: Two wrongs don't make a right. JAMA 270: 1737–1739, 1993
Kralewski JE: Predicting risk and utilization for health care populations. Workshop on perspectives in medical management. American College of Physician Executives, 1994
Lazarus A: Disputes over payment for hospitalization under mental health "carve-out" programs. Hosp Community Psychiatry 45:115–116, 1994
Lazarus JA, Sharfstein SS: Changes in the economics and ethics of health and mental health care, in American Psychiatric Press Review of Psychiatry, Vol 13. Edited by Oldham JM, Riba MB. Washington, DC, American Psychiatric Press, 1994, pp 389–413
Lundberg GD: United States health care system reform. JAMA 271: 1530–1533, 1994

McFarland B: Health maintenance organizations and persons with severe mental illness. Community Ment Health J 30:221–242, 1994

Mechanic D: Professional judgment and the rationing of medical care. University of Pennsylvania Law Review 140:1713–1755, 1992

Mechanic D, Ettel T, Davis D et al: Choosing among health insurance options: a study of new employees. Inquiry 27:14–23, 1990

Morreim EH: Balancing Act: The New Medical Ethics of Medicine's New Economics. Boston, MA, Kluwer Academic Publishers, 1991

Pellagrino ED: Rationing health care: the ethics of medical gatekeeping. J Contemp Health Law Policy 2:23–45, 1986

Relman AS: The health care industry: where is it taking us? N Engl J Med 325:854–859, 1991

Relman AS: What market values are doing to medicine. Atlantic Monthly, March 1992, pp 99–106

Relman AS: Medical practice under the Clinton reforms. N Engl J Med 329:1574–1576, 1993

Relman AS, Reinhardt U: An Exchange on For-Profit Health Care: For-Profit Enterprise in Health Care. Washington, DC, National Academy Press, 1986, pp 209–223

Rodwin MA: Medicine, Money, and Morals: Physicians' Conflicts of Interest. New York, Oxford University Press, 1993

Sabin J, Daniels N: Determining "medical necessity" in mental health practice. Hastings Cent Rep 24:5–14, 1994

Safran DG, Tarlov AR, Rogers WH: Primary care performance in fee-for-service and prepaid health care systems. JAMA 271:1579–1586, 1994

Sharfstein SS: Assessing the outcome of managing costs: an exploratory approach, in Psychiatric Treatment: Advances in Outcome Research. Edited by Steven Mirin. Washington, DC, American Psychiatric Press, 1991

Thompson DF: Understanding financial conflicts of interest. N Engl J Med 329:573–576, 1993

Wolf SM: Health care reform and the future of physician ethics. Hastings Cent Rep March–April 1994, pp 28–41

Section IV
The Future for Psychiatry in Organized Systems of Care

CHAPTER ELEVEN

Paradigms, Preemptions, and Stages: Understanding the Transformation of American Psychiatry by Managed Care

Alan A. Stone, M.D.

The Four Paradigms

Many disciplines including medicine, philosophy, economics, law, and political science compete to offer guidance on health policy. Using a cross-disciplinary perspective, Elhauge has described four overlapping paradigms emerging from this mix: the professional, the moral, the political, and the market paradigm (Elhauge 1994). Each paradigm offers an approach to decision making in health policy, but the paradigms conflict and overlap. These paradigms may be somewhat arbitrary, but they make intuitive sense as systematic ways of thinking about the cost and benefits of managed care in psychiatry. The professional paradigm focuses on standards of care based on clinical and scientific evidence; the moral paradigm focuses on the individual's right to health care and the provider's ethical duties and responsibilities; the political paradigm focuses on legislation, interest groups, governmental regulation, and centralized controlling agencies; and the market paradigm is about economic competition, productive efficiency, accommodating consumer preference, and achieving allocative efficiency. The premise of this chapter is that organized psychiatry has focused insufficient attention on the market paradigm and that managed care's transformation of medicine

---

Special thanks to Duncan C. MacCourt, J.D., for research and editorial assistance and for his thoughtful dialogue.

as practiced in the United States can be understood only as the product of relentless market forces.

Certainly the "wisdom" of managed care constraints has often been debated as though it were a question to be resolved primarily on professional grounds (i.e. within the professional paradigm). For example, critics have complained that managed care violates professional standards of care in ways that are harmful to patients (Avorn 1984; Levinsky 1984; Stone 1985). The National Alliance for the Mentally Ill subscribes to this critical view:

> Perhaps the most serious risks we face in this transition time are the continuing incentives to under-recognize, under-diagnose, and under-treat serious and persistent mental illness in systems that are still driven almost entirely by cost-containment. Further, the acute care model that has been the core of most managed care systems fails to recognize the comprehensive and long term nature of services and treatments needed by persons with schizophrenia, manic depressive illness, and other severe mental disorders. (Flynn 1994)

In response, managed care's defenders have replied that their protocols eliminate harmful and unnecessary care while establishing more effective treatment plans that confer greater benefits at lower prices. Defenders claim, sometimes eloquently, that they are providing better care and not just cheaper care (American Psychiatric Association 1991). Thus the professional paradigm debate has often been framed in terms of clinical experience and scientific double-blind studies of efficacy (i.e., how would competent practitioners treat this disorder). Unfortunately, almost all of the evidence offered in this debate is anecdotal, and, because outcome studies and efficacy evaluation are still in the process of development—particularly in psychiatry—this important debate will take decades to resolve (Krupnick and Pincus 1992; Stone 1990). Nonetheless, while the debate continues, so do the relentless cost-cutting measures. This demonstrates that the sweeping changes in psychiatric care have at least as much to do with economic forces as they do with the careful application of new scientific efficacy studies to an improving clinical practice (Grogan et al. 1994; Kuttner 1995).

Managed care has also been debated by psychiatrists on the high ground of the moral paradigm. Critics have expressed concerns about managed care's interference with both the confidentiality of the doctor-patient relationship and the patient's autonomous choices. Utilization reviewers have been impugned for making medical decisions on self-interested and unethical grounds (American Psychiatric Association 1991). Psychiatrists and other practitioners have been told that they have a basic ethical obligation to advocate on behalf of their patients when managed care restricts necessary treatments (Appelbaum 1993). In response, the advocates of managed care have dismissed or downplayed these criticisms by attributing them to the self-interests of fee-for-service providers greedily milking the cash-cow of third-party health insurance. Or they have insisted that fee-for-service mental health practitioners have failed to consider their moral responsibility for the "communal interests" of a society that can no longer provide unlimited resources to health care (Sabin and Daniels 1994). These moral/ethical arguments continue to go unresolved, and no doubt the debate will last at least as long as the debate over scientific efficacy (Dougherty 1992).

But while the experts debate just and ethical solutions to the quandary of society's limited resources, it should be noted that the fastest growing segment of managed care is the for-profit-sector (Iglehart 1994b). That sector brings a profit margin mentality to the health care quandary. Health care businesses are currently spending millions of dollars to organize regional, capitated health plans and to advertise them in the national and local media. This means that profit-maximizing stakeholders are extracting or expecting to extract large profits from the health care market as they reduce costs. At the same time, in their competition to enroll members, aggressively marketed managed care plans are raising consumer expectations by promising personalized care and benefits that can never be delivered (Emmanuel 1993; Fox et al. 1995). Again this demonstrates the thesis of this chapter, namely that powerful economic forces are working to change American health care, along with any putative moral or altruistic endeavor on the part of promoters to protect the public commons and to husband society's resources.

Certainly, within the political paradigm, all health care providers, including organized psychiatry, have played an active role in attempting to educate and influence government regulation and cost control. Organized medicine and other health care providers, though not always successful, are renowned for their lobbying efforts and their sophistication about the political paradigm. Ironically however, as argued in this chapter, the legislation that unleashed managed care, the Employment Retirement Income Security Act (ERISA), made its way through Congress in 1975 by a process that gave provider interest groups no opportunity to exert their influence. Indeed the full significance of ERISA was to become apparent only a decade later.

ERISA by no means provides the entire explanation for the emergence of managed care. However, it shifted the regulation of health care from the public sector to the private sector, the natural domain of the market discipline paradigm. This shift was exactly what advocates of the market discipline paradigm would have wanted.

Many health care policy experts independently recognized the conflicts between paradigms described by Elhauge. For example, Thurow, an economist, had emphasized the importance of resolving the moral and ethical paradigm questions before attempting to achieve market paradigm solutions (Thurow 1984).

However, the most important and interesting paradigm conflicts were between advocates of finding solutions within the political paradigm (e.g., government reform of health care) and those urging government deregulation to permit market paradigm solutions. Experts on each side of this dispute recognized that both regulation and competition were necessary; the disagreements were about how much of each was needed and in what order.

Government Regulation Versus Market Solutions

During the 1960s and 1970s, federal and many state governments favored what is called command and control regulation to contain the soaring costs of health care—for example, careful region-by-region health planning to control capital expenditures that were thought to accelerate the inflation of health care costs (Furrow et al. 1991).[1] But

---

[1] In light of these new regulatory schemes, hospitals had to justify the building of new facilities to accommodate equipment such as computerized axial tomography (CAT) scanners or surgical transplant facilities and obtain a certificate of need (CON) before starting construction (Furrow et al. 1991).

market discipline advocates complained that these governmental regulations prevented innovation, protected inefficient and outmoded facilities, and promoted bureaucratic red tape and political corruption (Havighurst 1988). Command and control regulation, these critics argued, was anticompetitive and counterproductive in light of the market discipline/economic paradigm, which advocated free market competition in health care similar to that in other industries (Havighurst 1988).

In addition, advocates of market discipline challenged the medical profession's leadership of the health care industry, claiming that business-trained specialists and entrepreneurs were better suited than medically trained physicians to make cost-effective capital allocations and to manage such a vast industry. One influential article argued that the favored not-for-profit structure of most hospitals was a case of wolves in sheep's clothing (Clark 1980). The author saw the not-for-profit hospital as perhaps geared to maximize physicians' incomes at the expense of other cost considerations (Clark 1980). Many market discipline economists either implicitly or explicitly shared this view, believing that physicians controlled the demand for their services as well as the supply. As a result, the argument went, the existing fee-for-service incentives of American medicine had to be changed. Prescient health economists favored competing capitated systems (Sprinkle 1994).

Advocates of a more competitive market in the 1970s focused their criticism on the AMA's principles of ethics for physicians as being protectionistic.[2] They looked to the Federal Trade Commission and the antitrust laws for legal artillery. The AMA had for many years insisted that the doctor-patient relationship was sacred. They objected to commercial interests or any third party that might intrude on the doctor's judgment or control the doctor's treatment decisions. These concerns were specifically embodied in the AMA's principles of ethics, one of which prohibited physicians from contracting in any manner that might "tend to interfere with or impair the free

---

[2] As sociologist Paul Starr has emphasized, this attack on the AMA reflected a convergence of liberal patient's rights advocates and conservative free market advocates who were united against the hubris of the medical profession (Starr 1982).

and complete exercise of his medical judgment and skill or tend to cause a deterioration in the quality of care." Another of the AMA's ethics principles prohibited physicians from soliciting patients, for example, by advertising (American Medical Association v Federal Trade Commission 1980). In 1979, the Federal Trade Commission (FTC) held that the AMA's enforcement of these two ethical principles constituted a conspiracy to restrict competition, and a federal court agreed (American Medical Association v Federal Trade Commission 1979). For example, the AMA's Maryland affiliate had determined that closed panels of doctors—an essential building block of managed care—violated the free-choice ethic (American Medical Association v Federal Trade Commission 1979). And according to the FTC, the ethical principle prohibiting advertising and solicitation had been "restrictively applied to . . . HMOs and other prepaid group practice plans" (Weller 1983). In its decision, the FTC forced the AMA to abandon these and many similar practices that had been based on interpretations of the ethical code. This case effectively ended organized opposition to managed care and helped set the stage for what was to follow: corporate control of medical care under various managed care strategies.

The election of President Reagan in 1980 brought to federal health care policy a rejection of command and control regulation and the adoption of a deregulatory, procompetitive approach. The tilt was real even though procompetitive health policy experts shared the general wisdom that some regulation would be needed (Furrow et al. 1991; Health Care Study Group 1994). For-profit health care enterprises, which had flourished since 1965 with the passage of Medicare and Medicaid, now became stronger players in what had been an industry dominated by not-for-profit hospitals and health insurance operating under the not-for-profit umbrella of Blue Cross & Blue Shield. Entrepreneurs, MBAs, and lawyers began to replace physicians in leadership roles as economic competition transformed the health care market. For the 12 critical years between 1980 and 1992, the federal government favored the market paradigm approach to health care and market discipline solutions reached by economic competition (Furrow et al. 1991; Health Care Study Group 1994). This tilt toward the free market is illustrated by the comments of one Reagan-appointed federal judge in an antitrust case involving the exclusion of a "willing provider" hospital from a newly established Blue Cross & Blue Shield preferred provider network:

> Competition is a ruthless process. A firm that reduces cost and expands sales injures rivals—sometimes fatally. The firm that slashes costs the most captures the greatest sales and inflicts the greatest injury. The deeper the injury to rivals, the greater the potential benefit. These injuries to rivals are byproducts of vigorous competition, and the antitrust laws are not balm for rivals' wounds. (Ball Memorial Hospital v Mutual Hospital Ins. 1986)

It was in this ruthlessly competitive economic atmosphere that managed care emerged as the dominant force, promising to control the allocation decisions of physicians while holding down costs and respecting the bottom line.

Managed Care and "Medically Necessary"

Much of pragmatic health policy under the professional standards paradigm comes down to a struggle over how to interpret the words *medically necessary* found in statutes and health insurance contracts (Hirschfeld 1992). Before managed care, the physician decided by his or her own standards of care what was medically necessary within the benefit limits. Managed care is a system of hierarchical or "top-down" controls over the meaning of "medically necessary." In the early stages of managed care, this was done by external utilization review. Under later stage capitated systems, the plan either selects professionals who are identified as conforming to the plan's definition of medically necessary, and/or the plan has a set of constraints, incentives, or even a protocol that micromanages costly medical decisions. This top-down control has been particularly evident in psychiatric care. The American Psychiatric Association, like other professional specialty associations, has responded to these top-down controls by producing practice guidelines to reflect a consensus for higher standards of care (American Psychiatric Association 1993). Managed care protocols and professional practice guidelines therefore can be understood as competing interpretations of what is medically necessary.

Independent physicians who lose their autonomy describe both protocols and guidelines as cookbook medicine.

Psychiatry has always been the stepchild in health care coverage, and despite a great deal of political rhetoric against discrimination, all public and private health insurance contracts have been legally permitted to limit mental health benefits. Managed care has further limited these unequal mental health benefits by routinely determining that covered treatments are not medically necessary (e.g., the insurance contract may provide for 30 days of inpatient hospitalization, but the managed care utilization reviewer [UR] will decide that only 5 days are medically necessary). Managed care by similar tactics has had the same cost-cutting impact across the board on health care services without explicitly limiting benefits. This concealed rationing is a critical feature of its acceptability and impact on health policy and health politics.

Elected officials face daunting choices in health politics. Either they must increase and/or redistribute the tax burden, or they must somehow regulate in order to control cost. Explicit rationing to control costs, however, means denying benefits to an identifiable group of patients; this creates a special interest group hostile to elected officials and raises difficult legal/ethical questions of discrimination. These problems are illustrated in the much discussed and controversial Oregon Plan, which seeks to ration health care among those eligible for Medicaid through a system of prioritizing medical conditions.[3] Although conceived as a way to control escalating Medicaid costs while providing efficient and needed medical care, the Oregon Plan has recently been challenged under the Americans with Disabilities Act (Astrue 1994; Flanagan 1994). In contrast, managed care seductively promises to control costs without explicitly denying any medically necessary benefit.[4] Aware of this difference, governors in several states are now looking to managed care and not to schemes like the Oregon

---

[3]Or. Rev. Stat. §§ 414.025–414.750 (1991).

[4]Such control has become urgent, for at the state level "Medicaid is now consuming almost half of new revenue dollars, squeezing out state expenditures for higher education, transportation and other social welfare expenditures, and forcing states, which generally cannot engage in deficit financing, to raise taxes." See, for example, Furrow et al. 1991.

Plan in order to control their Medicaid costs.[5] For example, in 1993 Tennessee received federal permission to cover an additional 500,000 indigent residents under Medicaid and to enroll all Medicaid recipients in managed care plans (Furrow et al. 1991). This shift of Medicaid to HMO managed care is clouded in recurring scandal and quality control problems dating back to California's initial foray into managed care in the 1970s (D'Onofrio and Mullen 1977; Meyer 1995).[6]

Similarly, there have been efforts to shift Medicare patients into managed care, specifically HMOs. Earlier attempts at this shifting also ended in scandal and criticism involving "questionable recruiting practices and difficulties in gaining redress through appeal or grievance procedures when services are denied" (Furrow et al. 1991). However, HMO recruitment of Medicare patients is once again being actively encouraged by advocates of reform, who believe that managed care will reduce or at least control costs and provide more comprehensive coverage (Margolis 1995).

Malpractice Liability and Managed Care

Interestingly enough, a great deal of psychiatry's managed care debate over professional standards and ethical-moral principles originated in interpretations of judicial opinions in lawsuits alleging malpractice by health plans and their peer reviewers (Appelbaum 1993). Typically the peer reviewer failed to approve the payment of a treatment that the responsible clinician considered "medically necessary." The much-cited *Wickline* case, for example, involved a refusal

---

[5] See memorandum in support of plaintiff's cross motion for summary judgment and opposition to defendant's motion to dismiss. Also see the alternative for summary judgment, *National Association of Community Health Centers v. Shalala and Oregon, Tennessee, Hawaii, Rhode Island, Ohio, Delaware, and Missouri*, case no. 1:94CV01238 (HHG), July 27, 1994, p. 14; the alternative states that 4 states have instituted statewide managed programs; 2 additional states will implement similar programs in early August 1994; 5 states have applications pending for similar managed care programs; and 11 states are currently preparing to request approval from the federal government for similar programs.

[6] New complaints about Medicaid managed care programs in Florida and California could signal major problems nationally in the shift of Medicaid to managed care.

to extend the hospital stay of a patient who had suffered serious complications after major vascular surgery (Wickline v State 1986). *Wilson,* another much-discussed case, involved a psychiatric patient who committed suicide after external peer reviewers set payment limits on his length of stay in a private hospital (Hughes v Blue Cross of Northern California 1990; Wilson v Blue Cross of S Cal 1990).

The *Wickline* and *Wilson* cases fathered an extensive literature on the treating physician's duty to advocate for his or her patient and suggested that the health plan or the peer reviewer might, under certain circumstances, be liable (Appelbaum 1993). One of the underlying assumptions of these cases seemed to be that the burden of legal liability could be shifted onto the health plan by the treating physician's advocacy on behalf of his or her patient. However, these cases on which so much ink has been spilled are quite exceptional (Sweede v CIGNA Healthplan of Delaware 1989; Teti v U.S. Healthcare, Inc. 1989). Most health plans and their peer reviewers, as will be described in the next section, have been insulated from legal liability by state and federal law. Even more important, utilization review and all of its cost-cutting incentives have been internalized by providers as managed care has matured into capitated alternative delivery systems that combine the fiscal and the treatment functions. The *Wickline* and *Wilson* cases are therefore less instructive as a legal matter and more misleading as a practical matter than they seemed at the time. Indeed, they may have been a distraction from the more important market discipline considerations that were relevant to the growth of managed care.

ERISA: The Federal Statute That Changed American Health Care

Although psychiatrists may not have focused enough on the market discipline/economic paradigm, they were among the first medical specialists to feel the economic impact of private sector regulation by managed care. The rest of medicine has now caught up. John Iglehart, the *New England Journal of Medicine*'s premier health policy journalist, reported "the gathering panic among many physicians who are losing patients to managed care plans" (Iglehart 1994a). He was describing the frantic lobbying efforts of the AMA and other physician specialist groups like psychiatry to protect their fee-for-service private practice as the U.S. Congress considered the ill-fated Clinton Health Plan. The President's plan would have expanded the role of managed care in an effort to achieve market discipline. But unlike his Republican predecessors, President Clinton wanted to create new governmental agencies, called alliances, and new government command and control regulation of various kinds to constrain the market (Blumstein 1994; Yarmolinsky 1995). The President's plan went down to defeat, partly because the health care landscape was already being radically transformed—if not reformed—by managed care health plans. This transformation was much to the satisfaction of corporate America, who, having long paid the piper, was now finally calling the tune.

In the previous three decades, major change was expected to come from the political paradigm. The medical profession and all of the other interest groups in the health care industry had expended millions of dollars and countless hours of effort attempting to shape national and state legislation (Starr 1982). As powerful and shrewd as these lobbies were, they had failed to identify and influence the drafting and enactment of the pivotal law that has facilitated the transformation of the health care industry through managed care. That critical federal statute was passed in 1976 as the Employee Retirement Income Security Act (ERISA) (Employee Retirement Income Security Act 1974). It was conceived with the best intentions by the staff of the late United States Senator Jacob Javits of New York, who was concerned about the fate of long-term employees of the Studebaker automobile company.[7] When that company went bankrupt, its employees' pension funds went with it. Senator Javits's federal legislation was designed to protect future workers from such a disaster. However, as ERISA made its way through Congress, health care benefits were added at the 11th hour to the pension protection bill almost as an afterthought (Mariner 1992), with consequences that would be fully appreciated only years later.

---

[7]Oral presentation by Eileen F. Serene, Esq., presented in Washington, DC, in 1994.

According to U.S. Census Bureau statistics, 85% of Americans are covered by some form of health insurance plan, provided in most cases by the government or their employer (Griner 1991; Raffel and Raffel 1989; Reynolds and Bischoff 1990). And for Americans possessing private health care insurance through their employee benefit plans, "ERISA is the governing statute" (Pataki, governor of New York v Travelers Ins. Co. 1995; Travelers Ins. Co. v Cuomo 1993). The language of ERISA—and the courts' interpretations of that language—therefore affect millions of insured Americans. But although ERISA was meant to protect employees, in operation it actually protects the employer's control over health care benefits. As one commentator has noted,

> ERISA allows employers to establish, modify, or cancel employee medical benefits plans without state or federal interference, so long as the plan's administration is consistent with ERISA's provisions. ERISA does not require that employers provide any specific health benefits, and courts lack the power to issue such mandates. As a result, employees covered by self-funded plans can be left without adequate health coverage. (Jameson and Wehr 1993)

Due to this permitted exclusion, employers may limit coverage of mental disorders and may even discriminate among conditions, excluding from coverage diseases involving high-cost treatments, such as Alzheimer's disease, schizophrenia, or even AIDS (Jameson and Wehr 1993). In other words, discriminating on the basis of a particular disability, be it physical or mental, was effectively permitted by the ERISA statute. For example, in one notorious case involving an ERISA plan, a federal court ruled that an employer could cut the medical benefits of an employee who had acquired AIDS and filed for benefits (McGann v H & H Music Co. 1991).

Because ERISA was intended to impose uniform federal standards on employee benefits, it contained a provision preempting "any and all state laws insofar as they may now or hereafter relate to any employee benefit plan."[8] A corporate employer's ERISA health plan therefore had to comply with federal law, but the state legislature

---

[8]ERISA § 5\14(a), 29 U.S.C. § 1144(a) (1982).

could not impose other state legal requirements on such ERISA plans. Nor could an employee go into state court to seek redress for some loss or injury caused by the ERISA plan. This preemption provision insulated the ERISA plan from malpractice claims. It is important to note that the Wickline and Wilson cases, previously described as being so central to the professional standards and ethics debate, were cases brought by patients in non-ERISA plans. In fact, Wilson, who committed suicide after his premature discharge from a psychiatric facility, not only had a non-ERISA plan, he was insured in another state and was mistakenly subject to utilization review in California where he was hospitalized.

The ERISA preemption of malpractice liability is most dramatically illustrated when we look not at mental health cases but at recent litigation on the denial of coverage of expensive cancer treatments. In 1993, a federal court considered the case of a patient who developed testicular cancer and was initially approved by his ERISA plan for autologous bone marrow transplant; however, the plan then denied the last stage of the transplant treatment, causing a delay that allegedly led to the patient's death (Spain v Aetna Life Ins Co. 1993). The court ruled that whatever the merits of the case might be, a wrongful death action against the ERISA plan administrator was preempted by the ERISA statute (Spain v Aetna Life Ins. Co. 1993). In contrast, that very same year, the estate of a woman who had been covered by a non-ERISA plan sued under somewhat similar circumstances and was awarded $12.32 million in compensatory damages and $77 million in punitive damages (Fox v Health Net of California 1993).

These examples dramatically illustrate the importance of ERISA protection. Unlike physicians who practice defensive medicine and hospitals that institute risk management because of malpractice liability, the managers of ERISA plans are in effect immune from suit. ERISA provisions allow only the recovery of benefits wrongfully denied to the patient and not compensation for the damages caused by the denial—the so-called consequential damages available in the typical malpractice lawsuit (Jameson and Wehr 1993).[9] In contrast to

---

[9]Note also that although a few courts in the past five years have allowed such damages, these were not malpractice cases, and this does not seem to be the dominant trend.

health insurance plans outside of ERISA—such as the plan from which the patient just discussed received a judgment totaling over $90 million—the ERISA statute neither allows recovery of extracontractual damages (e.g., damages for pain and suffering) nor punitive damages (Gaskell v Harvard Coop Society 1991; Jameson and Wehr 1993). This situation effectively prevents many patients from ever bringing suit against their plans, for contingency fee attorneys will not find it economically feasible to take on these patients' cases (Sanborn 1995).[10] In effect, the ERISA preemption clause acts as a shield protecting the health plans, leaving plan participants "betrayed without a remedy" (Degan v Ford Motor Co. 1989).

Despite these impediments to patients/plaintiffs, states were nonetheless still able to exercise some marginal control over ERISA plans under the so-called savings clause, which permitted the states to regulate health insurance companies under state insurance laws.[11] Under this clause, if a corporate employer purchased its health plan from an insurance company, it confronted the hurdle of state regulation (Metropolitan Life Ins Co. v Massachusetts 1985). Thus, if the state legislature, as happened in Massachusetts, passed a law requiring all health insurers to provide a certain minimum amount of outpatient mental health coverage, the insurance companies had to add those benefits to the health packages they were selling and pass the added cost on to the corporate purchaser.[12]

---

[10] However, note that in one class of cases—severe head injury leading to large hospital bills—the contingency-fee attorney may determine that his or her expected recovery makes litigation feasible.

[11] ERISA § 514(a)(2)(A), 29 U.S.C. § 1144(b)(2)(A) (1988).

[12] States also went further and used their authority under the insurance law "savings clause" in ERISA to regulate the hospital rates paid by different insurance companies. Commercial insurers selling coverage to corporations were charged a higher rate for hospital care, and those funds were used to cross-subsidize financially troubled health plans. For example, New York State required commercial insurers to pay a substantial tariff for their members' hospital care in order to support New York's financially troubled Blue Cross & Blue Shield. This is a form of command-and-control government regulation opposed by proponents of market discipline. Arguably, it forces efficient insurance companies to cross-subsidize inefficient ones. Although a federal appeals court agreed with this reasoning, the U.S. Supreme Court has recently up-

The Supreme Court's unanimous 1985 decision in *Metropolitan Ins. Co. v. Massachusetts* upheld the state statute that required insurers to include minimum mandated mental health benefits. But the decision also opened an escape hatch from state regulations.[13] In his opinion for the court, Justice Blackmun distinguished between plans that purchased insurance and therefore were part of the insurance industry—and thus were subject to state insurance regulation under the savings clause—and plans that self-insured (described in the opinion as "uninsured") and therefore were not considered to be part of the insurance industry.[14] Not surprisingly, many corporate ERISA plans used what turned out to be a huge escape hatch and became self-insured, avoiding state regulation by, for example, setting aside the equivalent funds and paying the health care costs themselves. In a 1987 case, the U.S. Supreme Court affirmed the Metropolitan distinction and upheld this self-insured ERISA plan exemption from state health insurance regulation (Pilot Life Ins. Co. v Dedeaux 1987).

The consequences of this preemption can be seen in the case of recent state-mandated coverage for psychiatric disorders. As the result of prolonged lobbying efforts, advocates for mental health convinced legislatures in three states, most notably Maryland, to amend their insurance laws and require equal mental health coverage (Legislative and Regulatory Developments 1994). However, the vast majority of citizens in these states are covered by self-insured ERISA and government plans. Those plans are exempt from the new state insurance law under the ERISA preemption clause or because they are federal programs like Medicare.

Since the passage of the Americans with Disabilities Act (ADA), there has been some hope that ERISA-based discrimination against health benefits for particular disorders could be curtailed. Indeed, there

---

held the New York statute, arguing that any other conclusion "would bar any state regulation of hospital costs" *New York State Conference of Blue Cross & Blue Shield Plans et al. v Travelers Ins. Co.; George E. Pataki, governor of New York v Travelers Ins. Co.; Hospital Association of New York State v Travelers Ins. Co.*, 514 U.S. 645, 115 S. Ct. 1671 [U.S., Apr. 26, 1995].

[13] Ibid.

[14] Ibid., 732, 747 (1985).

have been a few preliminary legal skirmishes by AIDS activists that, unfortunately for the cause of mental health benefits, have led to consent decrees or settlement agreements rather than useful legal precedents (Equal Employment Opportunity Commission (EEOC) v Allied Serv. Div. Welfare Fund 1993; EEOC v Tarrant Distrib., Inc. 1994; Estate of Kadinger v International Bhd. of Elec. Workers 1993; Mason Tenders Dist. Council Welfare Fund v. Donaghey 1993). There has also been some success using the ADA to challenge ERISA plans that discriminate against persons with mental disorders in their *disability insurance* coverage (Giliberti 1994). Although the ADA has encouraged New York's psychiatrists to support similar legal challenges against ERISA *health insurance* plans that discriminate by denying equal coverage to mental disorders (Psychiatric News 1995), legal experts are skeptical that such litigation will succeed (Giliberti 1994).[15]

Freed by these ERISA protections and the Supreme Court's holdings, American corporations, which had long been struggling with the rising costs of health benefits (Cowan and McDonnell 1993),[16] began to explore more aggressively the various cost-savings parameters of self-insured managed care (Burns and Thorpe 1993). While health care interest groups—including organized psychiatry—were lobbying Congress about government regulation, the health care industry began to be radically transformed by "regulations" issued by managed care health plans from the private sector.[17] The failure of the Clinton Health Plan left managed care as the dominant force for "reform" in American healthcare.

---

[15]Internal document, Council on Psychiatry and Law, American Psychiatric Association 1995 (not for publication).

[16]In 1965, American corporations spent 12.4% of their after-tax profits on health care; by 1991 that amount had risen to an astronomical 97.5%.

[17]Note that the "package of benefits" in the typical ERISA plan is the result of bargaining between management and labor. As previously mentioned, most of the major labor-management disputes in the past two decades have involved explicit attempts by management to reduce health insurance benefits or to shift more of the cost to employees. Managed care is obviously a preferable alternative to corporate America—just as it is to government—because it will reduce health care cost by nonvisible methods and thus avoid strikes.

The Role of Oligopsony Purchasing Power

The cost-saving regulation of provider allocations through managed care has gone hand in hand with what Ginzberg called the "monetarization" of health care that "set the stage for the explosive growth of for-profit medicine" (Ginzberg 1984). Ginzberg describes the transformation from charity, philanthropy, and free care to governmental subsidies, bond markets, and third-party payment including Medicare and Medicaid. With monetarization of the industry, the role of the for-profit sector has been far more important than just the size of its holdings would suggest. Its competitive buying and selling of assets, its creaming of the market, and its exploitation of opportunities created by faulty public policy have forced not-for-profit participants to pursue similar strategies in this money economy. A basic problem is that the for-profit participants skim off the paying, low-risk customers—the "cream"—and leave the low-paying and nonpaying, high-risk customers behind. The nonprofit sector cannot survive under those conditions; therefore, it must mobilize to compete for paying customers. The ethos of the health care industry has changed to emphasize these bottom line "monetary" considerations. A key factor in this new monetarized and competitive health care market has been oligopsony purchasing power.

Most psychiatrists have never heard of the word *oligopsony*, nor do they clearly understand the rather simple concept that describes the market conditions that empower the purchasers of health care.[18] Webster's defines oligopsony as "a market situation in which a few buyers control the demand from a large number of sellers" (G. & C. Merriam Co. 1965). Oligopsony and ERISA, two concepts alien to psychiatry,

---

[18] In 1992 this author submitted an article to a refereed psychiatric journal, discussing managed care and oligopsony purchasing power. Two of the four anonymous referees were particularly negative in rejecting this admittedly polemical critique. The rejected article argued that psychiatric standards of care were increasingly driven by monetary considerations rather than professional judgment and professional ethics. Oligopsony purchasing power was highlighted as the economic leverage available to managed care. One of the critical referees opined that he or she had never heard of the word *oligopsony* and that Stone had "invented a neologism." This retrograde mind-set about the basic economic language of markets is still widely prevalent in the psychiatric profession.

are the two blades of the scissors that are cutting up the fabric of the American health care system and changing the identity of psychiatry.

How Oligopsony Works

Even psychiatrists who do not clearly understand this critical market discipline concept have felt the impact of oligopsony purchasing power. A recent letter to the editor in the *Psychiatric Times* readily demonstrates this. The writer, a psychiatrist in private practice, lamented that the health insurance carrier for General Motors had unilaterally reduced reimbursements to physicians for professional services by 24% in 1995. The psychiatrist complained that when he went to his General Motors dealer and asked for an equivalent 24% discount on a 1995 Cadillac, he was sent on his way (Psychiatric Times 1995).

Life and the market are not always fair: The market difference between General Motors and the letter writer is that GM's health insurer was using its oligopsony purchasing power to impose a reduction in the market price paid for medical care. They could readily find many other physicians willing to accept their price. The single physician purchaser of a Cadillac had no comparable market power.

To understand oligopsony power based on this homely example, imagine that the American Medical Association organized a luxury car-buying plan and approached General Motors on behalf of all of its 50,000 members who were considering the purchase of a new Cadillac or some other GM luxury car in 1995. The AMA Plan might ask for a 24% discount on the purchase price of 50,000 Cadillacs and be given it. Furthermore, if the AMA approached all of the comparable domestic and foreign luxury automobile manufacturers to discuss the same potential 50,000-car purchase, they might find that somewhere they were able to get an even better discount price. Realize that each of the sellers of luxury automobiles who does not make the 50,000-car sale will lose a share of the 1995 market (i.e., the AMA members who, absent the group purchase, would have bought their automobiles from one of the other manufacturers). By organizing its members into a purchasing group and limiting their choice of an automobile, the AMA plan would be using oligopsony power in much the same way as do many managed care health plans. The AMA might even be able to tell General Motors how they wanted their cars built.

In the era of fee-for-service care, millions of individual patients subsidized by health insurance went around purchasing health care from providers. Now the tables have turned, and a small number of health plans go around purchasing health care from hundreds of thousands of providers. These plans use oligopsony purchasing power.

This health plan oligopsony purchasing power works best in regions of the country where there is an oversupply of medical beds or professional services. Managed care has perhaps unintentionally helped to "create" an oversupply by stringent utilization review standards and therefore has been better able to exploit its market power. Consider the case of the private psychiatric hospital, the institution that was among the first to feel the impact of managed care. All hospitals, in order to survive financially, need to maintain a certain occupancy rate, for example 65% occupancy of beds. Below that so-called census, the hospital, with its fixed costs and overhead, loses money.

When managed care's utilization review standards cut the median length of stay (LOS) in the hospital for a psychiatric patient from three weeks to one week, the average hospital needed three times as many patient admissions each year to maintain its previous census. During the 1980s, psychiatric hospital occupancy rates dropped from more than 70% to less than 50% as the result of managed care (Carpi 1995). Desperate for more admissions, all of the psychiatric hospitals in a given geographical area were eventually competing for more referrals. Furthermore, because managed care imposes more stringent utilization review criteria for admission, the available pool of potential hospital patients had simultaneously been shrinking. As a result, hospitals with large bed capacities and high turnover of patients with shortened LOS needed a constantly increasing market share of the shrinking pool in order to maintain their break-even census. This situation was true for all types of hospitals; faced with these pressures, over 800 hospitals throughout the country have closed since 1980 (American Hospital Association 1993).

Any managed care health plan with a large number of potential referrals thus could come to the hospital and demand a discounted hospital price because it possessed enormous market power. The struggling hospital had a choice between an empty bed producing no income and a full bed producing a discounted payment, for example, 75% of their usual daily rate. At the same time, all of the other managed care plans were attempting to strike similar, low-price bargains with these hospitals. Indeed, over the past few years, many large managed care plans have attempted to obtain what has been called "most favored nation status" with hospitals and other providers: They want the hospitals with which they contract to guarantee that their plan will be given the lowest rate the hospital will give to any plan (Crew and Steele 1988).

As one might expect, hospitals try to resist the leverage of this bargaining power. One obvious tactic is for all of the hospitals in a given market to get together and agree to the minimum rate they will accept. This tactic, however, runs afoul of the antitrust laws as anticompetitive collusion (Adams 1989/1990; Vita et al. 1991). Another tactic that hospitals can employ when faced with oligopsony purchasing power is to try to establish their own health plans by joining with physician groups and insurers to form integrated provider networks (Bazzoli et al. 1995). Hospitals, some experts believe, are ideally suited to lead these efforts because of their financial and management resources (Bazzoli et al. 1995). But all of the other stakeholders—physicians, medical schools, group practices, and so on—are also jockeying to control the emerging delivery system as they realistically worry about the concomitant loss of power and market share. Simply put, physicians are recognizing that either they will manage the American health care system, or they will be managed by it.

All of these integrated delivery systems create potential antitrust violations that must be guarded against when the plans are organized. The industry is changing so rapidly that it seems even the U.S. Justice Department is somewhat uncertain about policy. Some critics charge that federal antitrust enforcement has been so unpredictable and inconsistent that predicting which provider-hospital agreements will run afoul of antitrust enforcement guidelines has become notoriously difficult (Bazzoli et al. 1995; Vistnes 1995). As a result, the ultimate structure of the newer integrated delivery systems remains in doubt. But the trend is toward plans that combine the fiscal and provider functions in vertically organized systems.

Despite the uncertainty, antitrust law is a major concern to the stakeholders in the reorganizing health care market. Similarly, federal regulations dealing with Medicare and Medicaid fraud and abuse are crucial in reorganization. These regulations penalize compensation for patient referrals (e.g., kickbacks—that is, paying a primary care physician to send patients to a group psychiatric practice)[19] and therefore may apply to intrahealth network referrals where the referring physicians have an economic interest in the health plan (Baumgartner 1994).[20]

These antitrust and referral regulations are extremely complicated, but experts agree that they have a disparate impact on physician-providers (Baumgartner 1994; Bazzoli et al. 1995; Homer 1994). The opportunities to organize and exercise health plan oligopsony power have certainly been disproportionately seized by business entrepreneurs. The control of networks of providers has been detailed by *Managed Care Digest:* By 1992 insurance companies owned 42% of all preferred provider organizations; independent investors owned 24%; and 7% were owned by physician/hospital organizations (Merriam Merell Dow 1993). Only 4% were owned by physicians or medical groups (Merriam Merell Dow 1993). These figures demonstrate a major concern of organized medicine today: Unless these antitrust and fraud provisions are amended, business managers rather than physicians will dominate the future provision of all health care. And these managers will be primarily concerned with one thing—the bottom line.

---

[19]42 U.S.C.A. § 1320a-7b.

[20]Although the Comprehensive Physician and Ownership Referral Act of 1993 exempts qualified HMOs from the prohibition on physician referrals, some observers worry that the act might affect physicians in joint ventures established to service managed care plans. Consider, for example, the operation of the typical physician/hospital organization (PHO), which is designed to facilitate contracts between participating physicians and managed care entities. One commentator notes that such contracts might be interpreted as creating prohibited compensation arrangements between the physicians and the hospital because the PHO costs and funding typically would be "absorbed by the hospital system that made the managed care contracts available to the physicians" (Homer 1994). Similarly, it has been argued that each of the practice support services provided by management service organizations (MSOs), for example, space, equipment, personnel, and so on, could create prohibited financial arrangements if tied to referrals or not supplied at market rates (Baumgartner 1994; Homer 1994).

The managed care industry has begun to experience a trend that affected hospitals earlier. For-profit HMO chains are buying up not-for-profit HMOs to expand their market shares rapidly (Stein 1995). The purchase of a not-for-profit HMO, like a not-for-profit hospital, poses interesting questions: Who should get the money? Who decides on an appropriate price? Typically, the state attorney general will have oversight of the transaction. This shift to the for-profit form is being followed by many of the stakeholders in health care, including giants like California Blue Cross & Blue Shield. This for-profit shift fulfills the program of market discipline advocates skeptical about the not-for-profit model. This trend has nothing to do with the professional, moral, or political paradigms. It can be understood only in light of the market paradigm.

The market forces just described have made the plans both profit and not-for-profit, the new power brokers of the health care industry. These plans combine the fiscal and the provider function, and many are controlled by health insurance companies. Huge commercial insurance companies now market themselves as care-giving providers and are seeking to expand their control of the market. As a consequence, all of the other healthcare stakeholders—medical schools, hospitals, and physicians—are competing to organize and control their own health plans. Various corporate structures are being devised to maximize the interests of each competing stakeholder.[21] Psychiatrists and other specialists are struggling to find a place in some network because they confront a shrinking demand for their services. Despite the protean nature of these evolving structures, it is possible to describe the sequence of changes in managed care as occurring in four stages. Based on their impact on the psychiatric practitioner, these stages are 1) fee-for-service care with external peer review, 2) horizontal networks to organize mental health providers and to contract selectively with managed care health plans, 3) vertically orga-

---

[21]A recent innovation is the "physician-friendly" managed service organization, which, in contrast to hospital controlled MSOs, is majority owned by the physicians it serves. A valuable discussion of such "physician-friendly" managed service organizations appears in Bond: Pro-physician MSOs: a winning managed care strategy, HealthSpan, July/August, 1993, p 3.

nized carve outs of mental health care, 4) carve-ins reintegrating mental health care in one vertical health care plan.[22]

The first three stages track what are generally identified as the "major tools of managed care" that is, utilization review, negotiated discounts, and capitation (Furrow 1991). The step between negotiated discounts and full capitation is filled with elaborate partial compromises described here in terms of horizontal and vertical networks. Many of the second- and third-stage changes in the organization of health care have been the result of provider response and accommodation to the demands of managed care. The fourth stage is a futuristic description of the features of market consolidation (i.e., industry concentration) as they affect psychiatry in the long-term accommodation to managed care market forces.

The feature emphasized in each stage is not unique to that stage. HMOs are capitated, vertically integrated systems, but they have been part of American health care for most of this century.[23] Negotiated discounts were common early in this century (Starr 1982). And many forms of utilization review are certainly still with us. Thus one can cite many exceptions and overlaps in the features of these stages that are meant to be no more than "ideal types" in the Weberian sense.[24] There is some empirical/historical basis for each of the four stages, but they are described so as to highlight dominant features that are not unique. The driving conception of these stages is to highlight the market discipline paradigm that altered the flow of health care

---

[22] These stages roughly correspond to Saul Radovsky's personal account of the past three decades of American medical practice published in the *New England Journal of Medicine* (Radovsky 1990).

[23] The first HMO was established in California in the 1930s by the Kaiser Corporation to serve its employees. For a good overview of the establishment of the Kaiser Permanente health plan, see Starr 1982.

[24] In Weber's work, the concept of the ideal type " 'refers to the construction of certain elements of reality into a logically precise conception.' Such a construct is intended to focus attention on an abstracted version of certain descriptive characteristics, which can then be used for comparative, analytic purposes." Mark Neal Aronson, *Dark Night of the Soul: A Review of Anthony T. Kronman's The Lost Lawyer: Failing Ideals of the Legal Profession*, 45 Hastings L J 1379, 1382 (1994), quoting H. H. Gerth and C. Wright Mills, *From Max Weber: Essays in Sociology* (1958).

"upstream" from where the psychiatric profession was debating standards, ethics, and government reform of health care.

Stage 1

Many of the methods we now know collectively as managed care began as attempts to control costs in a predominantly fee-for-service market with payments by third-party indemnity and service benefit health insurers. They include more stringent claims review, various forms of utilization review, prospective payment (DRGs), second opinions for elective surgical procedures, co-payments by patients, and so on (Furrow et al. 1991). Some of these developments are more familiar to the rest of medicine than to psychiatry. All of them can be understood as attempts to control the allocative decisions of physicians.

For psychiatry, the most important aspect of managed care in stage one was the increasingly intrusive role of "fourth-party" utilization review, that is, the "outside scrutiny of physicians' medical decisions" (Morreim 1991). In this fourth-party conception, the covered patient is the first party, the provider is the second party, and the insurer or self-insured ERISA plan is the third party. The fourth party is the utilization reviewer (UR), a company retained by the third-party payer to monitor the quality as well as the cost of mental health care at the hospital-patient and/or doctor-patient levels (Morreim 1991).

An early, benign era of fourth-party utilization review that promised quality assurance as well as cost control inexorably gave way to URs who emphasized cost cutting. These fourth-party, typically for-profit URs represented the start up of a new type of business in medicine that would ultimately become managed care organizations (MCOs). They would make money not by providing care to patients but by acting as intermediaries to save the money of such third-party purchasers of health care as standard indemnity and service-benefit insurance plans and particularly ERISA plans.

Entrepreneurs—often mental health professionals themselves—could set up with very little capital investment a specialized company to do psychiatric utilization review for third-party payers. The URs' contractual arrangement with the ERISA plan or other third parties who retained them often included a contingency fee based on annual performance (i.e. the cost reduction they achieved in the insurer's mental health payments). These for-profit URs typically employed nurses or social workers backed up by psychiatrists to do the actual reviewing. These reviewers were trained to scrutinize claims and to require that any proposed treatment be justified as medically necessary—a justification measured by their newly established, cost-effective standards. The more the reviewers cut utilization, the more the UR company made.

Over time, utilization review shifted from retrospective to concurrent to prospective authorization; each shift increased the control of the utilization reviewer (Morreim 1991). Eventually it could be said that many URs were dictating the nature and duration of care—that is, how to treat as well as how much to treat.

Working with ERISA plans, utilization review contractors were protected by federal law from malpractice liability for the consequences of their decisions as previously described (Corcoran v United Healthcare, Inc. 1992; Gordon 1995; Varol v Blue Cross & Blue Shield 1989). Although URs not protected by ERISA remained subject to malpractice liability,[25] if some serious harm to a patient occurred as a result of inadequate care or care improperly denied, the legal case against the treating psychiatrist often seemed much stronger than the case against the fourth-party nurse reviewer or the utilization review contractor.[26] As a result, URs could control providers without being overly concerned about the legal consequences.[27]

---

[25] See, for example, *Wilson v. Blue Cross*, 271 Cal Rptr 876 (Cal App 2 Dist 1990). However, at least one commentator has expressed concern that, as current health care standards "evolve toward an accommodation of the economic values inherent in rationing decisions," URs may begin to successfully apply cost control as a defense against malpractice actions. In this scenario, a non-ERISA malpractice claim against a UR may fail if the UR's review practices meet community standards (Schessler 1992).

[26] This was certainly the consensus of an APA subcommittee of the Commission on Judicial Action, of which the author was a member. We reviewed cases with a view to the possibility of litigating these issues despite the impediments of ERISA.

[27] Efforts by physicians to impose legal consequences include model legislation that would make utilization review the practice of medicine, thus subjecting URs to malpractice liability and disciplinary intervention by boards of medical examiners. See McCormick (1995) discussing *Blue Cross & Blue Shield of Arizona v. Arizona Board*

The UR companies that focused on mental health services were certainly not the first group of for-profit psychiatric entrepreneurs to set up as businesses. In 1965, the passage of Medicare and Medicaid had set off a chain reaction of for-profit enterprises in health care. Notable were the nursing home chains out of which emerged the giant of for-profit medicine, Humana, Inc. Alongside these developments came the for-profit psychiatric hospitals and their chains, followed by substance abuse treatment centers and their connected chains. There is no doubt that these for-profit mental health care providers were geared specifically to the profitable benefit packages of third-party payers. The most transparent example was one for-profit chain that in the same facilities provided long-term renal dialysis covered by Medicare and short-term psychiatric hospitalization covered by standard third-party service and indemnity insurance.[28] In the capitalist jungle of free-market competition, these URs were the natural enemies of the benefit-oriented for-profit providers.

With ERISA protecting them, the "lean and mean" URs had no natural enemies, but they soon discovered that fourth-party utilization review over time becomes cumbersome, labor intensive, and after the first few years, much less remunerative on the contingency fee basis. To remain profitable in stage II, each UR therefore needs both to reduce its utilization review expenses and find other ways to service its third-party clients. And despite their protestations, health care providers must adapt to these same stringent standards or take themselves out of the market for managed third-party payment.

Stage I From a Market Perspective

This first stage of fourth-party utilization review was, and still is, the subject of many criticisms on the grounds of professional standards and ethics. However, from the perspective of the market discipline paradigm, it looks quite different. Third-party payers like Blue Cross

---

of Medical Examiners, citations omitted, which held that a state medical board had jurisdiction over medical decisions made by an HMO medical director who denied coverage for gallbladder surgery.

[28]Information derived from author's personal knowledge.

& Blue Shield certainly had limited and unequal mental health benefits. But to the extent there was coverage, third parties simply collected premiums from employers and made out checks to providers doing little or nothing to control cost or ensure quality. As Joseph Califano, the former secretary of Health, Education, and Welfare (now Health and Human Services) complained, health insurance companies had no incentive to control costs (Califano 1986).

The Blue Cross & Blue Shield bureaucracy was typically paid some previously negotiated percentage of the premiums they had collected. Therefore, the more health care costs and premiums escalated, the more money came in, and the more Blue Cross & Blue Shield grew and prospered. At the same time, the Blues' corporate boards were dominated by representatives of the providers they were paying.[29] From the market discipline point of view, Blue Cross & Blue Shield was a typically bloated, not-for-profit operation under the control of the medical profession who should have been kept at arm's length. Secretary Califano strongly agreed and introduced regulations to end provider domination of health insurance boards (Califano 1986). The basic principle of sharply limiting provider control of health care institutions has dominated federal regulation ever since (McCarthy and Weinstein 1994).

The real economic urgency to control costs came from the large corporations who were paying the premiums that kept escalating and from the federal government, which had to find more tax dollars to pay for health care (McNeil 1988).[30] To these purchasers, utilization review companies seemed the first evidence of a businesslike market control on health care costs. And whatever else the fourth-party UR claimed to be, it indisputably was a business being driven by a market, and it brought market forces to bear on mental health care. By the standards of the free market advocates, this was an admirable demonstration of how market discipline should work to control costs.

---

[29] As Radovsky described the situation, half of the board were physicians, and the other half were people they knew (McNeil 1988; Radovsky 1990).

[30] McNeil writes that health care premiums rose 25% a year in the 1980s, and retiree medical costs rose from 2% of payroll to approximately 5% from 1973 to 1978. Ibid. (citations omitted).

Stage II

The second stage of managed care in psychiatry is characterized by discount pricing and selective contracting. As mentioned earlier, fourth-party utilization review had helped to create an oversupply of both beds and service providers—an oversupply that paved the way for oligopsony purchasing power in the second stage. The first most visible example of the use of oligopsony purchasing power came with the emergence of a new form of health care organization, the preferred provider organizations (PPOs). California was an early hotbed of PPOs, and although it had different labels, the arrangement rapidly spread across the country (Furrow et al. 1991). The basic organizational strategy behind the PPO is to create a health plan "network" through *selective contracting* that limits the panel of specialists and the choice of hospitals available to plan enrollees. PPO enrollees who go outside the plan for treatment from a physician or hospital not on the panel must pay a substantial additional copayment. The plan organizers therefore negotiate with specialists and hospitals in order to obtain discounted fees for both services and beds in exchange for referrals exclusively to those hospitals or specialists, who become the plan's "preferred providers" (Loue 1993).

The market dynamic of this bargaining process is impressive to watch. Fearful of losing market share, hospitals and specialists who have been complaining about low reimbursement rates and trying to raise fee-for-service prices are suddenly prepared to offer lower prices. The most impressive early example took place outside psychiatry. The administrators of the California Medicaid program, MediCal, had endlessly struggled with providers over hospital rates and fees for professional services (Crocker 1994; Kennedy 1984; Perkine 1989). Now they turned the tables and asked hospitals to submit competitive bids to participate in a PPO (selective contract arrangement) for the same patients they had been complaining about under preexisting market conditions (Gittler 1984). Suddenly, a low-paying MediCal patient seemed better to many of these providers than a vacant bed. The concern about losing patients took hold even more strongly among specialty practitioners. In some geographical areas, medical specialists—including psychiatrists—were willing to pay an entry fee to be a listed provider in a PPO network that would pay them a discounted rate.[31]

The organization of PPOs was one of many new networking arrangements, most of which at this juncture were horizontally integrated. Psychiatrists were already working in group practices, a form of horizontal integration that rapidly increased. Many new, loosely organized groups of mental health providers emerged, seeking to enter into selective contracts with PPOs. Both for-profit and not-for-profit hospitals organized horizontally to take advantage of marketing, shared administrative costs, and large group purchasing. For-profit psychiatric hospital chains expanded, merged, and multiplied. Specialty substance abuse, eating disorder, and adolescent facilities proliferated in response to new insurance coverage. The industry spun off new corporate entities: management services, continuing medical education, marketing, clinical laboratories, and so on. A basic economic strategy was to move profitable functions away from the nonprofit hospitals to the domain of the for-profit entrepreneur. What Relman called the "Medical Industrial Complex" (Relman 1980) had become a presence in psychiatry as well as the rest of medicine. Horizontal integration and the growth of for-profit chains was one of its manifestations.

As demonstrated by the success of the PPOs, the advantages of oligopsony purchasing power were quickly and sometimes painfully obvious to third-party health insurers like Blue Cross & Blue Shield. PPOs allowed more aggressive health insurers to offer lower, more competitive premiums to ERISA plan purchasers because they were paying discounted prices to providers. Although the pace of events varied in different regions of the country, these and other market pressures causing loss of market share and loss of low-risk patients were driving many Blue Cross & Blue Shield organizations into the red (Brown 1991; Sapolsky 1991).

This second stage of managed care has been colorfully described as "the sleeping giants awaken." The sleeping giants were the third-party health insurers like Blue Cross & Blue Shield, who suddenly had to

---

[31] See Plaintiff's Verified Complaint—Class Action at 22, *Schiffer, M.D., et al. v. Blue Cross & Blue Shield of Mass., Inc., and Bay State, Inc.*, Mass. Sup. Ct. (No. 94–1563-B).

wake up and play a more active role in the monetarized and increasingly competitive health market (Furrow et al. 1991). But the awakened giants were no more active than the aggressive managed care organizations (MCOs) in mental health and substance abuse who offered to be insurers' agents in creating lower cost, preferred provider networks in addition to performing utilization review. The MCOs therefore grew and prospered by combining their UR role with a new and powerful role of selective contracting with providers at discounted prices. Recall that the UR could now to a large extent dictate standards of care in the process of applying prospective and concurrent utilization review. Relying on their oligopsony purchasing power, these MCOs in stage II took their business to providers who would agree explicitly or implicitly to follow their guidelines at a discounted fee.

Market Disciplines Effects in Stage II

In this second stage, preferred provider organizations and selective contracting mark the abandonment of the gentleman's agreement convention originally established by not-for-profit Blue Cross & Blue Shield. This agreement, in which every licensed physician and hospital could bill third-party payers, had been reached during the early days of the Blues as a response to the introduction of direct-service "single-hospital" plans, in which a hospital contracted with a group of patients to supply care for a set rate (Starr 1982).[32] In contrast to such single-hospital plans, local hospitals jointly developed "community-wide" plans that provided "free choice" among hospitals and physicians (Starr 1982).[33] Faced with these two competing models of health plans, the American Hospital Association encouraged the development of community-wide plans due to the feeling that the single hospital

---

[32]The first of such single-hospital plans was developed by the Baylor University Hospital in 1929, when it agreed to supply to 1,500 school teachers up to 21 days of hospital care a year in exchange for a payment of $6 per teacher. Ibid.

[33]This not-for-profit form was premised on community-based premiums, that is, pooling the high and low risks, and its provision of free choice was an effort to enlist the cooperation of not-for-profit hospitals and skeptical physicians in a broadly based effort. Ibid.

plans resulted in "competition among hospitals, and interference with the subscriber's freedom of choice and the physician's prerogatives in the care of private patients" (Starr 1982).[34] A similar approach soon followed for Blue Shield payment of physicians.[35] In addition, provider control of the boards of Blue Cross & Blue Shield was also part of that original accommodation, often written into the state laws enabling the Blues (Califano 1986; Starr 1982).

The collapse of the gentleman's agreement that had prevented competition and the proliferation of plans that either limited patients to a fixed panel or charged them extra to go outside the plan made it increasingly important for providers to be part of a plan. The urgency increased as these plans caused preexisting patterns of referrals to break down. For example, the general practitioners who had previously referred many of their patients to psychiatrists might now be part of a PPO that referred only to the psychiatrists within the PPO network. Private psychiatric hospitals left out of the referral network were in equally difficult straits.

Although there were considerable variations in the psychiatric markets across the country, MCOs prospered in stage II. Critics of these developments, including some of the mental health professionals employed as utilization reviewers, worried that the MCOs were, in their pursuit of cost savings, being transformed from businesses founded on a health care ethos to bottom-line corporate entities.[36] These corporate-culture MCOs were able to squeeze still more dollars out of providers

---

[34]Ibid., 297–298. Starr notes that by 1939, as a result of intense lobbying by hospital and medical leaders, "twenty-five states had passed special enabling acts for hospital service plans" (i.e., Blue Cross plans. Ibid., 298).

[35]However, although the AHA encouraged the establishment of Blue Cross plans, the American Medical Association vigorously opposed the Blue Shield plans' coverage of physicians' fees as an intrusion on the doctor-patient relationship and, it should be noted, as a control upon physicians' incomes. Dominated by general practitioners, the AMA grudgingly accepted Blue Shield only after the surgeons who saw the financial advantages outmaneuvered the general practitioners. The gentleman's agreement of universal participation in medical insurance coverage therefore evolved as a complex accommodation between the many conflicting interests on the provider side (Starr 1982).

[36]Personal conversation with utilization review employee.

and take their share. They selected cost-effective providers by their bottom-line standards and established the mental health PPO network at discounted prices, and they continued their role of utilization review. And because an oversupply of mental health providers exists, those chosen to be part of the network are beholden to the MCOs.

Note the possible consequences to providers in these circumstances of oversupply: If psychiatrists advocate, criticize, and make trouble for the MCO, the psychiatrists and/or their hospital can be eliminated from the preferred provider network. The pressures on psychiatrists to keep silent and go along with the managed care program are therefore enormous. Furthermore, because the MCOs enjoy ERISA immunity, no strategy of shifting legal responsibility onto their shoulders will work.

As described earlier, federal fraud and abuse regulations concentrate on physician referrals that could be construed as involving illegal kickbacks.[37] However, because MCOs are not considered health care providers, they are not subject to these regulations (Homer 1994). As a result, some MCOs have developed a sophisticated prospective review and referral system, wherein the enrolled patient desiring psychiatric care must first dial a toll-free number and speak to a mental health care professional, often a nurse, who will screen the call and then refer the patient for treatment.[38] Although proponents of this procedure claim it allows for efficient patient management, in practice this system clearly permits the MCO to channel the patient away from disfavored member psychiatrists and toward compliant mental health practitioners.

Because MCOs are profitable and have relatively low capital start-up costs, they attract competition. Because their main product is cost reduction, the very existence of competitors forces the MCOs to bargain even harder with health care providers over price. And because individualized utilization review is expensive, the MCO also needs to lower its review costs in order to maintain its profitability. These cost reductions

---

[37] See supra notes 19–20 and accompanying text.

[38] Formal Demand Letter from Daniel L. Goldberg, Esq., to Edward J. Dailey, general counsel and chief legal officer, Blue Cross & Blue Shield of Massachusetts, Inc. (Feb. 14, 1994), citing Bay State Health Care Guide 19 (letter on file at Dr. Alan Stone's office).

can be achieved by a variety of methods employing the MCO's referral leverage over providers to shift over to them most of the utilization review function. These methods will be discussed further in stage III.

The Market in Stage II and Professional Standards of Care

As external utilization review shortened the median length of stay, the style of psychiatric hospital practice had to accommodate. Hospitals that wanted to be preferred providers found it necessary to adapt their entire treatment approach. This contributed to the ongoing shift of hospital psychiatry toward rapid psychopharmacological interventions, short-term and symptom-focused psychotherapies and behavioral treatments, as well as a more biological emphasis in the biopsychosocial treatment model.

The transformation of psychiatric hospitals by these relentless economic pressures in stage II made most of the much publicized Osheroff–Chestnut Lodge debate between the late Dr. Gerald Klerman and the present writer quite irrelevant and obviously misplaced (Stone 1990). We were debating in terms of the professional and moral paradigms: standards of care, informed consent, malpractice liability, and the role of psychoanalytic therapy in the treatment of a hospitalized patient. But in retrospect those paradigms were beside the point, for by the time the debate was published, the hospital's approach had already drastically changed. These changes were dictated as much by the market discipline paradigm described in this chapter as by conclusive double-blind scientific studies of efficacy. Driven by market pressures, the private sector simply could not wait for scientific answers before issuing managed care regulations.

Contributing to the recent growth of managed care and carve-out MCOs has been the computerization of medical records, medical charges, and other medical information. Although discussion of computerized systems has often focused on the balance between their greater efficiency in storing and generating information and patient rights to privacy (Field 1994), the use of such systems has also markedly transformed both comprehensive utilization and peer review—a transformation that has allowed MCOs, hospitals, and health plans to develop databases containing profiles of individual physicians.

These profiles detail the manner in which physicians practice medicine, for example, their patterns of diagnosis, prescription, and treatment, and their utilization of medical resources, tests, and referrals. In other words, the profiles indicate how likely a particular physician may be to prescribe one form of treatment over another that may cost less. Using these computerized databases—and recently developed, specialized software—MCOs can select for their healthcare network psychiatrists and other providers who are cost effective by the standards of utilization review; conversely, those practitioners who are not cost effective are identified and deselected or prevented from participating in the health plan.[39]

All of the stakeholders involved in supplying psychiatric services are financially threatened by the formation of selectively contracted networks. This extends all the way from the individual practitioner to the prestigious departments of psychiatry in medical schools. Most disturbing, the MCOs have the market power to impose their requirements and exclude or deselect providers who do not accommodate. Across the board in medicine, physicians—particularly specialists—are desperate not to be left out of the network. The same is true for all of the other providers. Even medical schools, which traditionally have been financially dependent on their teaching hospitals, can be decimated by being excluded from selective contracting (Kassirer 1994).

Seeking to stop the market forces of stage II by government regulation, many of the guilds have gone to the state legislatures and sought

---

[39] Furthermore, as such databases develop, they will become more effective in performing this screening function. Many commentators now envision a national health information network that in the near future will electronically link our entire health care system. When established, such a system could allow MCOs to develop a national databank of physicians who are cost effective and those who are not. If each individual physician's computerized profile contains an evaluation of his or her cost effectiveness—or even the history of such review by MCOs that have examined his or her treatment records—the potential increases for an effective national screening of physicians. At the very minimum, it should be realized that the growing sophistication of computerized profiles has in stage II effectuated the MCOs' efforts to allocate patient care among "efficient" practitioners, and the future development of the national health care "infobahn"—the information superhighway—will allow further allocative decisions based on a psychiatrist's treatment history (Field 1994; Gobis 1994; Rotenberg 1995).

Paradigms, Preemptions, and Stages 221

the passage of "Any Willing Provider Laws" (Duffy 1994). And the AMA has proposed model state and federal statutes to guarantee participation in health care systems to any willing provider (AWP).[40] In effect, these efforts are an attempt to go back to the earlier described anticompetitive gentleman's agreement (i.e. the arrangement wherein any licensed provider can be part of the healthcare network).

These AWP laws face legal and political obstacles. Passage of legislation would be opposed by corporate America and proponents of managed care.[41] Federal AWP legislation would in effect amend ERISA, a possibility that would open a Pandora's box of conflicting interest groups. Unless some such drastic political paradigm solution is found, fee-for-service practice will be further curtailed in the vertically organized systems of stage III.

Stage III

Perhaps the most instructive example of how the market compels health care reorganization is the now familiar prospective payment scheme of "diagnosis related groups" (DRGs) introduced by the Reagan administration to control the cost of Medicare part A (Furrow 1991). Prior to the implementation of DRGs, Medicare had paid hospitals on a cost plus basis: The higher the hospital's daily rate, and the more tests ordered, procedures completed, and days the patient spent

---

[40] Patient Protection Act, American Medical Association, May 1994 (on file with Dr. Stone); Patient Protection Act: State Version, American Medical Association, Department of State Legislation, June 1994 (on file with Dr. Stone).

[41] How ERISA's preemption and savings clauses will apply to individual state "any willing provider" laws is still an unsettled legal question. One federal court has held that the ERISA preemption does not apply to Virginia's "any willing provider" statute: *Stuart Circle Hospital Corporation v. Aetna Health Management*, 955 F. 2d 500 (4th Cir. 1993), cert. denied, 114 S. Ct. 579 (1993). However, a Connecticut court has recently found that state's Managed Care Act of 1994 to be preempted by ERISA, "insofar as it was claimed that the law was violated by CIGNA Healthcare of Connecticut Inc., in unilaterally removing physicians from its preferred provider panel." Gordon (1995) citing *Hollis v. CIGNA Healthcare of Connecticut, Inc.*, Conn. Super. Ct., docket no. CV705357; *Napoletano v. CIGNA Healthcare of Connecticut, Inc.*, docket no. CV705358, 12/5/94 (3 HLR 1835).

in the hospital, the larger would be the hospital bill the government had to pay.

Under the prospective payment system of DRGs, the government instead paid the hospital a fixed lump sum amount set in advance and based primarily on the patient's condition requiring hospitalization (e.g., so much money for treatment of a heart attack and not a penny more). Thus the fewer tests, procedures, and so on ordered and the shorter the length of hospital stay, the larger the hospital's surplus of the DRG payment.

With the advent of DRGs, the hospitals' and the doctors' economic interests diverged in a significant way. Operating within a fixed prospective payment scheme, hospitals for the first time had an economic necessity to monitor their medical staff's allocative decisions. Doctors who ordered many expensive procedures and prolonged hospitalizations now became a financial drain on the hospital rather than an asset. The hospital had to pursue utilization review diligently in order to avoid spending more than its DRG reimbursement. As a result of these new economic incentives operating upon hospitals, Medicare had much less need for costly external utilization review. DRGs required the hospital to internalize that burden and to make the process stringent.[42]

While DRGs were not applied to psychiatric hospitalizations, the further developments that characterize stage three in psychiatry and lead to vertical integration can be seen in the following related example. The managed care organization (MCO) of a major ERISA health plan sees the virtues of prospective payment systems and wants to go beyond stage II organization. The MCO will therefore approach a psychiatric hospital as a potential preferred provider of acute psychiatric hospitalization services. The MCO offers to pay the hospital a negotiated amount to be responsible for supplying all of the necessary treatment for that acute episode. This system is even more cost effective than the lump-sum DRG payment just described, for the hospital

---

[42] However, hospital care provided by physicians is paid from a different source, Medicare part B. Doctors and hospitals were not in direct conflict about who got how much of the lump sum payment. That would happen in this third stage under MCO incentives.

must share the acute episode payment with its doctors. If the hospital refuses, the MCO is prepared to exert its oligopsony purchasing power and offer another competing psychiatric hospital the chance to become the MCO's preferred provider.

Empirical studies by health economists have demonstrated that working together under this kind of lump sum incentive, hospitals and doctors can significantly reduce costs (Shortell et al. 1994). The cost reductions come both from further reductions in length of stay and the more limited use of more expensive specialist services. For example, whenever possible a less expensive psychiatric nurse will supply the medically necessary service rather than a more expensive psychiatrist. This can be described as a *human economy of scale*.[43] Such human economies of scale inevitably mean that fewer psychiatrists are needed to deal with the same number of patients.

If it accepts such a lump sum acute episode arrangement, the psychiatric hospital will not only need to do its own utilization review—taking much of the MCO cost burden as the general hospital does for Medicare with DRGs—but in addition it will need to organize some form of physician-hospital organization (PHO). It will have to select from within its staff the fewer *necessary* doctors to provide the cost-effective services. This usually means that participating physicians are placed on a salaried basis (Shortell et al. 1994). The resulting corporate entity will be vertically integrated, for example, hospitals and mental health professionals.

Notice that the MCO acute episode proposal requires this vertical reorganization and forces hospitals and psychiatrists to agree to the value of each side's contribution. As Shortell et al. (1994) note, the formation of such a PHO requires commitment, leadership, and trust on the part of both hospital and physicians—a set of requirements that may not be easily achievable (Shortell et al. 1994). The stakes are high because some members of the staff have to be excluded from the PHO under these circumstances. This situation represents a dramatic trans-

---

[43]In economic parlance, economies of scale are those decreases in costs associated with an increase in production. In this case, by comparison, a similar human economy of scale occurs when a psychiatrist assisted by nurses can "produce" many more treatments—can treat more patients—at less cost.

formation away from the traditional hospital-psychiatrist relationship. The psychiatrist's value to the hospital now depends on the cost of his or her contribution relative to the amount budgeted by the MCO.

The HMO as an Example of a Capitated System. The key element of an HMO that will characterize the market changes in stage three is capitation, the joinder of the fiscal insurance function, and the completely vertically organized provider function. Such capitated systems seem to be the wave of the future in medicine and the hallmark of stage III.

The health maintenance organization is the first and most familiar example of capitation. In the simplest case, the HMO has available all health care services and provides for all of the health care needs of its members in exchange for an annual capitation payment, that is, so much per head, or in the current jargon, per "covered life" (Shortell et al. 1994). The HMO accepts the risk that it can operate within an annual budget determined by those aggregated capitation payments while meeting the needs of its membership (Furrow et al. 1991). Capitation therefore creates financial incentives for the HMO to control allocation decisions and to limit expensive tests, procedures, and treatments. At the extreme, the HMO has an incentive to give as little care as possible. These incentives under capitation are diametrically opposed to those of the "old world" of indemnity-based, fee-for-service medicine. The market discipline paradigm anticipates competition among such capitated systems for enrollees, as is occurring in stage II.

At present, approximately 50.5 million people—one fifth of the United States population—are enrolled in HMOs (Schear 1995). Because vertically organized health care systems often lack mental health services, the HMO may enter into a "carve out" arranged by an enterprising MCO. This means that the MCO will set up a network to provide all needed mental health care in exchange for a portion of the capitation payments. The MCO will in turn extract its broker's profit from the portion of the capitation fee allocated to mental health services. This kind of carve-out MCO arrangement has dominated stage III, although the HMO might in theory go directly to a provider group that had vertically organized and would accept the capitation risk. This latter arrangement will eliminate the MCO and dispense with the agent who played such a critical role in stages I and II (Shortell et al. 1994). And the MCO's services can be dispensed with in part because the need for stringent utilization review has to be internalized by any provider under capitation. Because the MCO has occupied a profitable niche, they will make every effort to contest this development.

The "would be" mental health service carve out that wants to compete with the MCO needs to offer the HMO a vertically organized, "one-stop shopping" partner who will provide all of the mental health and substance abuse needs of enrollees. The mental health partner of the HMO thus becomes responsible for providing all medically necessary mental health care, but not on a cost plus or negotiated fee-for-services basis. And like the HMO, it now combines the fiscal and provider function for all enrollees.[44]

In the real world there is an enormous overlap in the provision of mental health services between primary care physicians and psychiatrists. Approximately seven million prescriptions for psychotropic medication are written by primary care physicians for their patients, many of whom do not even recognize that they have a mental health problem (Olfson and Pincus 1994). In an HMO carve out with divided capitation between mental health and other providers, primary care physicians might have an incentive to refer these patients to the mental health side and let the carve-out partner bear the cost. In a similar manner, the mental health carve out might have an incentive to push all patients with somatic complaints to the medical side. Rules and agreements can be made to manage these problematic incentives, but the divided carve-out arrangement cannot entirely avoid them.

A horizontal network of psychiatrists and other mental health professionals providing only psychotherapy is not positioned to engineer a carve out. Neither is a geographically isolated psychiatric hospital and its staff. They will need to deal with an MCO middleman. At the very least, a capitated system needs a large group psychiatric practice capable of providing the full range of mental health and substance abuse services with access to in-patient and intermediate care facilities.

One of the candidates for a carve out without an MCO intermediary

---

[44] What the proper percentage of the capitation fee for mental health and substance abuse should be is something of a mystery and subject to negotiation.

might be a medical school department of psychiatry that already has access to all or most of the necessary ingredients for vertical organization, can form a PHO, and can outplace providers to cover the geographical area. However, capitation's economic incentives and its human economies of scale run counter to the traditions of excellence in teaching hospitals (Rogers et al. 1994). Either those costly traditions must be compromised, or the carve out is financially impossible. But the alternative of not doing the carve out means the continuing loss of the department's clinical income as the plans who "own" the patients send them elsewhere as described in stage II. Medical schools that refuse to accommodate to stages II and III managed care thus face devastating financial consequences as their teaching hospital beds empty.

The completed non-MCO carve out means, to quote the cartoon character Pogo's motto from the Vietnam era, "we have seen the enemy and they are us." The department of psychiatry—not the MCO—in the carve-out condition becomes the agent of all the stringent managed carve functions. Protocols, UR, micromanagement, computer profiles of cost-effective providers, stringent definitions of medically necessary: All have to be internalized. Most important for the profession of psychiatry, the carve out, even when it is a teaching hospital or medical school department of psychiatry, now operates under the burden of the human economy of scale incentives that have previously made many psychiatrists redundant in stages I and II.

The non-MCO carve-out department with its fixed capitation budget must now replace psychiatrists with psychologists, psychologists with social workers, and social workers with nurse practitioners whenever possible. Just like any other tight-fisted "insurer-provider" of health care, the carve out will have little interest in paying psychiatrists to do long-term psychotherapy. Operating under its capitation economic incentives, the carve out will offer long-term psychotherapy only when it must, and it will select the least expensive providers. Such treatment will be provided only when it clearly reduces the carve out's need for some more costly service such as in-patient psychiatric care. Cost-effective treatment and "medically necessary" will be redefined relative to the capitation budget rather than in terms of traditional standards of care.

The carve-out arrangement may entirely exclude the horizontal networks of psychotherapy providers who were organized in stage II unless they are essential in covering geographical regions. Because the department of psychiatry will be excluding from the carve out many of its own clinical faculty who have now become redundant, it will have a strong incentive to outplace them to obtain geographical coverage. And some distinguished academic psychiatrists will find the medical school that once deemed them indispensable now urging them to take early retirement.

The medical school department carve out competing over price with an MCO is unlikely to be able to cross-subsidize clinical research and teaching from capitation funding. Given the changed style of capitated HMO practice, departments of psychiatry will inevitably be teaching their students and house officers a quite different approach. As a result, the next generation of psychiatrists will learn a different role. The role played by the psychiatrist in a carve-out arrangement will emphasize *medical training*, primarily diagnosis and biological treatments. Those are the psychiatrist's basic value-added functions. Experienced psychiatrists can also provide various kinds of supervision. Anything else the psychiatrist provides can be obtained by the carve out at a lower price from a nonmedically trained professional who costs less.

It must be emphasized that these drastic changes in psychiatry and psychiatric training will not be based on clinical experience and scientific outcome studies. The role of psychiatrists and the content of residency training in psychiatry will be changed because of the changing health care market. The relentless economic pressure dictated by capitation incentives leads to every possible human economy of scale. The psychiatrist's future added value to a carve out responsible for covered lives will come from his or her medical training.

Psychologists and social workers who had "shadow priced" up the fee scale ladder of psychiatrists in billing third-party payers will be back-pedaling or risk being shut out.[45] In a stage III mental health

---

[45] "Shadow pricing" refers to the practice of setting treatment fees by referring to the fees currently being charged for other existing treatments of similar conditions, regardless of the inherent cost of providing those different treatments. For example, cardiologists have set their fees for cardiac catheterization by referring to their fees for coronary bypass surgery. Fees for catheterization therefore are high because they "shadow," or reflect, the high fees for bypass surgery.

carve out, professional guild and price distinctions will collapse toward the lowest cost provider as dictated by the human economies of scale. All providers of nonmedical services will become fungible to the carve out, and all will be paid less. Psychiatrists who prefer to do psychotherapy can expect to be paid the same salary as the generic provider.

One thing is very clear: A vertically organized carve out will need many fewer psychiatrists than were needed in stage I or stage II. Stage III of managed care may mean that up to 50% of the existing psychiatric labor force will become superfluous in some geographic areas.[46] Similar projections have been made for other medical specialties and for hospital beds.[47]

Capitation, as previously noted, is no longer limited to the basic HMO. Any health plan can be capitated, and one can predict that in the future, many more will try to institute capitated regimes due to the undoubted, competitive financial advantages. Studies in general medicine indicate that, even after cost savings achieved by UR—such as shortened LOSs—integrated capitation can achieve further cost reductions of 35% per member per month in the area of hospital care and a reduction of 16% in specialist care (Shortell et al. 1994).[48]

The capitated, mental health carve out and the growth of other vertically organized networks will isolate further the fee-for-service private mental health practitioners. Unless they can survive on a carriage trade of patients who are prepared to pay out-of-pocket, they will become extinct. Some psychotherapists undoubtedly will survive outside of health plans, as it is estimated that 45% of outpatient mental health services is now paid out-of-pocket (Olfson and Pincus 1994).

---

[46] Personal experience based on confidential meetings at Boston hospitals regarding projected teaching hospital utilization within the greater Boston area.

[47] Ibid.

[48] Studies indicate that integrated, capitated plans can reduce the length of stays from 6.6 days to 5.1 days in one month; can reduce LOS "for the top ten . . . DRGs from five days to four days after six months;" and can reduce LOS for coronary artery bypass surgery from 10 days to 6.5 days in one year (Shortell et al. 1994).

Stage IV

The basic feature of this stage is the predicted reintegration of mental health services into vertically organized systems (i.e., the "carve-in" idea) and industry concentration. For example, the non-MCO carve out of a department of psychiatry in stage III will become a "carve in" when the whole medical school, or its teaching hospital, is involved in organizing its own PHO capitated health plan. Such an arrangement that eliminates both the separate HMO health plan and the MCO is what many medical school teaching hospitals would prefer as they try to organize to compete for patients. In the "carve in,"[49] the department of psychiatry has rejoined the department of medicine and surgery, putting all of health care back together and sharing one capitation payment. They may offer their own health plan, become a regional branch of a national health plan, or work out a variety of other capitated packages. In theory, this will both mitigate the carve-out problem of separately capitated departments foisting patient care off on each other and eliminate the role of the MCOs and their intermediary's piece of the health care dollar.[50] The carve in, the basic feature of stage IV, is therefore considered a positive development by some academic psychiatrists. However, the long-term fate of psychiatry as a

---

[49] There are several versions of the carve-in idea now being discussed, but the basic idea involves a reintegration of mental health care into health care.

[50] The most recent development of capitated organizations moving in this way can be seen in the advent of "direct contracting," in which a large employer bypasses both the HMO and the MCO to contract directly with health care providers "on a capitated or predetermined price basis" (Schoen and Falchek 1994). Typically, such large businesses control substantial patient volume, particularly in small to mid-sized communities that may be serviced by only a handful of hospitals (Schoen and Falchek 1994). These employers can therefore utilize their oligopsony purchasing power in a manner similar to that discussed earlier. Because they control a significant percentage of the potential patients for each hospital, the employer can negotiate substantial reductions in health care costs, effectively forcing the hospital to agree to deliver a one-stop package of health care at a fixed cost. This means the hospital must vertically organize with its physicians, for example, into a physician-hospital organization. Note that this new direct arrangement is not confined to "company towns" with smaller populations and fewer hospitals: As one commentator notes, "there are some signs that direct contracting is becoming a reality in urban areas" as well (Schoen and Falchek 1994).

thriving, growing specialty in this ultimate stage of vertically organized capitated health care looks bleak over the long run.

As previously described, paying a percentage of the capitation fee for carved-out mental health services becomes inefficient due to cost shifting incentives. If stage IV produces all-encompassing carve ins as expected, past experience provides no reason to believe that psychiatry and mental health services will receive a fair share of the health care budget.

If we look at how cost saving occurs under current arrangements, we can perhaps see the outlines of the future. At the core of most capitated schemes that are gaining market share is the much advertised primary care physician, functioning as gatekeeper. It is much less well advertised in managed plan marketing that the primary care physician is insulated from providing direct, "hands-on" primary care as the result of a system of nurse practitioners, physician extenders, and other less costly providers who actually treat the patient. Such a situation is dictated by the current need for human economies of scale. Many of the initial contacts and tasks of the primary care physician are assumed by these lower-paid nonphysicians. So too, many of the tasks of medical specialists are assumed by the lower-paid primary care physicians. In the framework of these gatekeeper plans, most mental health services in the future will be provided by these primary care personnel (general practitioners, nurse practitioners, physician extenders, etc.) who are the cost-saving core of the plan. The medical part of the medically trained psychiatrist will shift as much as possible (e.g., diagnosis and drug prescription) to the primary care physician. The nonmedical part of psychiatry will be provided by nurse practitioners and other less well paid professionals working in the integrated medical setting rather than by more expensive psychiatrists, psychologists, or psychiatric social workers.

This version of the fourth stage carve in requires even fewer psychiatrists than stage III; furthermore, their expertise will primarily be neurobiological, and they will function as supervisory consultants who deal directly with only the most complicated cases. Once again this new and highly limited role will not necessarily be dictated by science or professional wisdom. It will once again be the result of the relentless economic pressure that requires human economies of scale so as to maximize the cost savings of a fully capitated health system.

In such a fully developed system, some projections suggest, less than 10% of the currently practicing psychiatrists would be necessary (Grinfeld 1994).[51]

Experts in health policy seem to agree that market forces will lead to increasing horizontal consolidation of most of these new vertically organized health care providers. Major cities will have several vast capitated plans. Plans will horizontally regionalize and nationalize. Medical schools and teaching hospital PHOs may not be able to control, or even lead, these vast organizations. Medical schools that created strong HMOs able to grow will eventually be dwarfed by them.

The long-term result will be competing health care behemoths similar in many ways to the "big three" in the automobile industry. There is an interesting irony in this industry concentration that has been noted by health policy experts: Unleashing the free market in the name of competition will have led to massive organizations that in the end resemble the monopolies or oligopolies that are the bane of free-market economists (Weil 1995). Because they are providing essential services, they will become quasi-public utilities (Weil 1995). The public utility is typically a monopoly providing essential services to captive consumers and therefore requiring close governmental regulation. We will therefore eventually find our way back to the political paradigm.

Conclusion

From the point of view of the psychodynamic psychiatrist who specializes in fee-for-service psychotherapy, each stage of managed care has further narrowed his or her career horizons. But subsequent stages have narrowed the career horizons for the whole profession of psychiatry as they have for all other medical specialists. Psychiatrists can endlessly debate these events within the professional standards and moral/ethical paradigms. However, one need only look at other medical specialties that are undergoing the same drastic changes to see that our parochial debate is downstream from where the relentless

---

[51] Citing discussion of one health care model that requires only 5,000 psychiatrists nationwide.

market is at work. It is extraordinary to watch the quality of American medicine deteriorate as the stock market value of managed health plans reach new highs. Only if we understand private sector regulation under both ERISA and the market paradigm will we comprehend how that is possible.

References

Adams CM: Nonprofit hospital mergers: proceed with caution. Cumberland Law Review 20:719–767, 1989/1990
American Hospital Association: Hospital data center report. 1993
American Medical Association: Patient protection act. May 1994a
American Medical Association: Patient protection act, state version. June 1994b
American Medical Association v Federal Trade Commission, 94 FTC 701 (1979), modified and enforced 638 F2d 443 (2d Cir 1980), aff'd mem, by an equally divided court, 102 S Ct 1744 (1982)
American Medical Association v Federal Trade Commission, 638 F2d 443 (2d 1980) (citing AMA Principles of Medical Ethics § 7)
American Psychiatric Association: Ethics in Managed Care Conference: Transcript Summary. Washington, DC, American Psychiatric Association, 1991
American Psychiatric Association: Practice guidelines for major depressive disorder in adults. Washington, DC, American Psychiatric Association, 1993
Appelbaum PS: Legal liability and managed care. Am Psychol 48:251–258, 1993
Aronson MN: Dark night of the soul: a review of Anthony T. Kronman's the lost lawyer: failing ideals of the legal profession. Hastings Law Journal 45:1379–1382, 1994
Astrue MJ: Pseudoscience and the law: the case of the Oregon Medicaid rationing experiment. Issues Law Med 9:375–386, 1994
Avorn J: Benefit and cost analysis in geriatric care: turning age discrimination into health policy. N Engl J Med 310:1294–1301, 1984
Ball Memorial Hospital v Mutual Hospital Ins, Inc., 784 F2d 1325 (7th Cir 1986)
Baumgartner MR: Physician self-referral and joint ventures prohibitions: necessary shield against abusive practices or overregulation? Journal of Corporation Law 19:313–335, 1994

Bazzoli GJ, Marx D Jr, Arnould RJ, et al: Federal antitrust merger enforcement standards: a good fit for the hospital industry? J Health Polit Policy Law 20:137–163, 1995

Blumstein JF: Health care reform: the policy context. Wake Forest Law Review 29:15–45, 1994

Brown LD: Capture and culture: organizational identity in New York Blue Cross. J Health Polit Policy Law 16:651–670, 1991

Burns LR, Thorpe DP: Trends and models in physician-hospital organization. Health Care Manage Rev 18:7–20, 1993

Califano J: America's Health Care Revolution: Who lives? Who dies? Who pays? New York, Random House, 1986, pp 40–128

Carpi J: Managed care pushes psychiatric care outside of hospital walls. Clinical Psychiatric News, February 1995, p 12

Clark RC: Does the nonprofit form fit the hospital industry? Harvard Law Review 93:1416–1489, 1980

Corcoran v United Healthcare, Inc., 965 F2d 1321 (5th Cir 1992)

Cowan CA, McDonnell PA: Business, households and governments: health spending 1991. Health Care Financ Rev 14:227–249, 1993

Crew E, Steele JJ: Some antitrust issues for managed care systems: joint ventures, most favored nation clauses and staff privileges. Practising Law Institute Commercial Law and Practice Course Handbook Series 471:309–326, 1988

Crocker B: California moves to manage Medicaid. Psychiatric Times, June 1994, p 54

Degan v Ford Motor Co., 869 F2d 889 (1989)

Diamond C, et al: Access to specialty care (letter). N Engl J Med 332:474, 1995

D'Onofrio CN, Mullen PC: Consumer problems with prepaid health plans in California: implications for serving Medicaid recipients through HMOs. Public Health Rep 92:121–134, 1977

Dougherty CJ: Ethical values at stake in health care reform. JAMA 268:2409–2412, 1992

Duffy JF: Managed care systems shut doors to MDs. Psychiatric Times, September 1994, p 1

EEOC v Allied Serv. Div. Welfare Fund, no. 93–5076 (CD Cal 1993)

Elhauge E: The moral paradigm for allocating health care resources. Paper presented at Harvard Law School Faculty Workshop, April 4, 1994

Emmanuel EJ: Managed competition and the patient-physician relationship (Sounding Board). N Engl J Med 329:897–898, 1993

Employee Retirement Income Security Act of 1974, Pub L no. 93-406, 88 Stat 829 (codified as amended in various sections of IRC (West 1988 & Supp 1990) and 29 USC §§ 1001-1461, 1988)
Equal Employment Opportunity Commission v Tarrant Distrib, Inc., no. H-94-3001 (SD Tex, October 11, 1994)
ERISA § 514(a), 29 USC § 1144(a), 1982
ERISA § 514(a)(2)(A), 29 USC § 1144(b)(2)(A), 1988
Estate of Kadinger v International Bhd. of Elec. Workers, 63 Empl Prac Dec (CCH) 42,783 (D Minn 1993)
Field RI: Overview: computerized medical records create new legal and business confidentiality problems. HealthSpan 11:3-7, 1994
Flanagan TB: ADA analysis of the Oregon health care plan. Issues Law Med 9:397-424, 1994
Flynn LM: The impact of managed care. National Alliance for the Mentally Ill (NAMI) Advocate 16:1, 1994
Fox v Health Net of California, Calif Superior Court (Riverside) no. 219692 (12/23/1993)
Fox PD, Rice T, Alecxih L: Medigap regulation: lessons for healthcare reform. J Health Polit Policy Law 20:31-48, 1995
Furrow BR, Greaney TL, Johnson SH, et al: Health Law: Cases, Materials, Problems, 2d Edition. St. Paul, West, 1991, pp 683-694
G & C Merriam Co.: Webster's Seventh New Collegiate Dictionary. Springfield, MA, G & C Merriam Co., 1965
Gaskell v Harvard Coop Society, 762 F Supp 1539 (D Mass 1991)
Giliberti MT: The application of the ADA to distinctions based on mental disability in employer-provided health and long-term disability insurance plans. Mental and Physical Disabilities Law Report 18:600-603, 1994
Ginzberg E: The monetarization of medical care. N Engl J Med 310:1162, 1984
Gittler J: Hospital containment in Iowa: a guide for state public policymakers. Iowa Law Review 69:1263-1311, 1984
Gobis LJ: Protecting the confidentiality of computerized medical records. HealthSpan 11:11-13, 1994
Gordon MS: Managed care, ERISA pre-emption, and health reform—the current outlook. Bureau of National Affairs Health Law Reporter 4:630-634, 1995
Griner DD: Paying the piper: third party payer liability for medical treatment decisions. Georgia Law Review 25:861-922, 1991
Grinfeld MJ: Managed behavioral health care charts a new course. Psychiatric Times, July 1994, p 61

Grogan CM, Feldman R, Nyman JA, et al.: How will we use clinical guidelines? The experience of Medicare carriers. J Health Polit Policy Law 19:7–26, 1994
Havighurst CC: Health care, Law and Policy. Westbury, NY, Foundation Press, 1988
Health Care Study Group: Understanding the choices in health care reform. J Health Polit Policy Law 19:499–511, 1994
Hirschfeld EB: Should ethical and legal standards for physicians be changed to accommodate new models for rationing health care? University of Pennsylvania Law Review 140:1809–1816, 1992
Homer LC: How new federal laws prohibiting physician self-referrals affect integrated delivery systems. HealthSpan 11:21–31, 1994
Hughes v Blue Cross of Northern California, 245 Cal Rptr 273 (Cal App 1 Dist 1990)
Iglehart JK: Changing course in turbulent times: an interview with David Lawrence. Health Aff Winter, 1994a, p 65
Iglehart JK: The struggle between managed care and fee-for-service practice. N Engl J Med 331:63–67, 1994b
Jameson EJ, Wehr E: Drafting national health care reform legislation to protect the health interests of children. Stanford Law and Policy Review 5:152–175, 1993
Kassirer JP: Academic medical centers under siege. N Engl J Med 331:1370, 1994
Kennedy JJ: The Medicaid program: vague standards breed litigation. Social Security Reporter Series 6:963–998, 1984
Krupnick JL, Pincus HA: The cost effectiveness of psychotherapy: a plan for research. Am J Psychiatry 149:1295–1305, 1992
Kuttner R: Market forces are the wrong medicine for health care sickness. Boston Globe, February 27, 1995, p 15
Legislative and regulatory developments. Mental and Physical Disabilities Law Report 18:318–319, 1994
Levinsky NG: The doctor's master. N Engl J Med 311:1573–1564, 1984
Loue S: An epidemiological framework for the formulation of health insurance policy. J Leg Med 14:523, 1993
Margolis RE: Will funneling seniors into managed care reduce costs? HealthSpan 12:16–17, 1995
Mariner W: Problems with employer-provided health insurance: the employee retirement income security act and health care reform. N Engl J Med 327:1682, 1992

Mason Tenders Dist. Council Welfare Fund v Donaghey, no. 93-Civ-1154 (SDNY 1993)

McCarthy BJ, Weinstein T: Special strategies sidestep legal, regulatory obstacles to health care mergers and acquisitions. HealthSpan 11:7–20, 1994

McCormick B: When coverage decisions threaten care: utilization review becomes new medical board concern. American Medical News, February 20, 1995, p 1

McGann v H & H Music Co., 946 F2d 401, 408 (5th Cir 1991), cert. denied sub nom

McNeil JT: The failure of free contract in the context of employer-sponsored retiree welfare benefits: moving towards a solution. Harvard Journal on Legislation 25:213–273, 1988

Merriam Merell Dow: Managed Care Digest, HMO Edition. Kansas City, MO, Marion Merrell Dow, 1993

Metropolitan Life Ins. Co. v Massachusetts, 471 US 724, 105 S Ct 2380 (1985)

Meyer H: Quality problems could spell trouble for Medicaid HMOs. American Medical News, January 23–30, 1995, p 7

Morreim EH: Balancing Act: The New Medical Ethics of Medicine's New Economics. Dordrecht, Boston Kluwer Academic Publishers, 1991, pp 34–36

Olfson M, Pincus HA: Measuring outpatient mental health care in the United States. Health Aff 13:172–179, 1994

Pataki, governor of New York v Travelers Ins. Co.; Hospital Association of New York State v Travelers Ins. Co., 115 S Ct 1671, 1995 WL 238409 (US, Apr 26, 1995)

Perkine J: Increasing provider participation in the Medicaid program: is there a doctor in the house? Social Security Reporter Series 26: 846–919, 1989

Pilot Life Ins. Co. v Dedeaux, 481 US 41, 107 S Ct 1549 (1987)

Psychiatric News: Area 2 goes ahead with plans to sue employers with discriminatory coverage. Psychiatric News, March 17, 1995, p 1

Psychiatric Times, February 1995, p 3

Radovsky SS: U.S. medical practice before Medicaid and now—differences and consequences. N Engl J Med 322:263–267, 1990

Raffel M, Raffel N: The U.S. Health System: Origins and Functions. New York, Wiley; Media, PA, Harwal, 1989, p 239

Relman AS: The new medical industrial complex. N Engl J Med 303:963, 1980

Reynolds J, Bischoff R: Health Insurance Answer Book 2, 2nd Edition. New York, Panel Publishers, 1990

Rogers MC, Snyderman R, Rogers EL, et al: Cultural and organizational implications of academic managed care networks (Sounding Board). N Engl J Med 331:1374–1375, 1994

Rotenberg M: Review of health data in the information age: use, disclosure, and privacy. J Health Polit Policy Law 20:235–241, 1995

Sabin JE, Daniels N: Determining "medical necessity" in mental health practice. Hastings Cent Rep, November-December 1994, pp 5–14

Sanborn R: ERISA is prototype for pre-emption. National Law Journal, April 17, 1995, p 1

Sapolsky HM: Empire and the business of health insurance. J Health Polit Policy Law 16:747–760, 1991

Schear S: Shock treatment for a sick system. Bus Health, March 1995, p 30

Schessler CE: Liability implications of utilization review as a cost containment mechanism. J Contemp Health Law Policy 8:379–404, 1992

Schiffer, M.D. et al. v Blue Cross and Blue Shield of Mass, Inc., and Bay State, Inc., Mass Sup Ct (no. 94–1563-B)

Schoen EJ, Falchek JS: "Covenants not to compete" gain vital new importance in era of healthcare acquisitions. HealthSpan 11:3–10 January 1994

Shortell SS, Gillies RR, Anderson DA, et al: The new world of managed care: creating organized delivery systems. Health Aff 13:46–60, 1994

Spain v Aetna Life Ins. Co., 11 F3d 129 (9th Cir 1993)

Sprinkle RH: Remodeling health care. J Health Polit Policy Law 19:45–68, 1994

Starr P: The Social Transformation of American Medicine. New York, Basic Books, 1982

Stein C: HMOs approve merger. Boston Globe, April 12, 1995, p 49

Stone AA: Law's influence on medicine and medical ethics. N Engl J Med 312:309–312, 1985

Stone AA: Law, science, and psychiatric malpractice: a response to Klerman's indictment of psychoanalytic psychiatry. Am J Psychiatry 147:419–427, 1990

Stuart Circle Hospital Corporation v Aetna Health Management 955 F2d 500 (4th Cir 1993), cert denied, 114 S Ct 579 (1993)

Sweede v CIGNA Healthplan of Delaware, Inc., WL 12068 (Del Super Ct), 1989

Teti v U.S. Healthcare, Inc., Civ A nos 88–9808, 88–9822 (ED Pa 1989)

Thurow L: Learning to say no. N Engl J Med 311:1569–1572, 1984

Travelers Ins. Co. v Cuomo, 14 F3d 708, 711 (2nd Cir 1993), rev. by New York State Conference of Blue Cross & Blue Shield Plans et al v Travelers Ins. Co.
Varol v Blue Cross & Blue Shield, 708 F Supp 826 (ED Mich 1989)
Vistnes G: Hospital mergers and antitrust enforcement. J Health Polit Policy Law 20:175–190, 1995
Vita MG, Langenfeld J, Pautler P, et al: Economic analysis in health care antitrust. J Contemp Health Law Policy 7:73–115, 1991
Weil TP: Powerful networks could result in public utility-style regulation of heath care. HealthSpan 12:12–15, 1995
Weller CD: Antitrust, joint ventures and the end of the AMA's contract practice ethics: new ways of thinking about the health care industry. North Carolina Central Law Journal 14:3–32, 1983
Wickline v State, 192 Cal App 3d 1630, 239 Cal Rptr 810, review granted 727 P2d 753, 23 Cal Rptr 560 (1986), review dismissed, 741 P2d 613, 239 Cal Rptr 8095 (1987)
Wilson v Blue Cross, 271 Cal Rptr 876 (Cal App 2 Dist 1990)
Wilson v Blue Cross of S. Cal., 222 Cal App 3d 660, 271 Cal Rptr 876 (1990), review denied (1990), Cal App LEXIS 4574 (1990)
Yarmolinsky A: Supporting the patient (Sounding Board). N Engl J Med 332:602–604, 1995

CHAPTER TWELVE

The Identity of the Field in the Context of Changing Roles

John J. Boronow, M.D.
Steven S. Sharfstein, M.D.

Psychiatry today faces the greatest challenge to its professional identity since its inception. External economic and social forces have coalesced in such a way that the very rationale for the existence of the field has been challenged. These forces can be reduced to three major trends: 1) limited and shrinking resources for reimbursement, coupled with 2) a new mandate to provide more services to a broader spectrum of society, within the context of 3) a revolution in the delivery of those services and the allocation of those resources through the imposition of a free market model based not on the doctor-patient relationship but on "capitated lives," "health care alliances," and corporate entities competing for patients and dollars.

As we consider the future identity of the field, it is important to keep in mind that although these forces may dramatically affect the *praxis* of our profession, they do not directly bear on its essential medical/scientific *knowledge base*. The knowledge and therapeutics we have developed over the past 150 years remain intact, open to scientific challenge and improvement to be sure, but essentially invulnerable to economic and social forces. Our task is to consider how to protect and further psychiatry's scientific foundations in a transitional era where our own professional identity with regard to praxis is being redefined. Our thesis is that if the profession of psychiatry keeps a clear and articulate focus on its medical and scientific knowledge base, then a coherent and meaningful professional identity will survive the impact of the current social and economic forces that are transforming us.

The Biomedical Foundations of Psychiatry

What in fact constitutes the medical and scientific basis of our field? First and foremost, psychiatry is a branch of medicine. As such, it contains within it the general medical model of illness, the specific biopsychosocial model of behavior, and the Hippocratic doctor-patient relationship.

The Medical Model

Once in danger of being diluted or dispensed with altogether in psychiatry, the general medical model has reemerged as a defining element of the field in the last 20 years. The discoveries of biological psychiatry, which describe major mental illness in terms of the same genetic and pathophysiological processes that pertain to the rest of medicine, make the medical model lucid and acceptable even to the lay public. The medical model includes both a body of knowledge about the brain and behavior, and specific values. Among these values is a sense of professional *virtue* (Dyer 1988). By virtue we mean values such as honesty and dedication, as well as directives about the physician's appropriate conduct, such as maintaining confidentiality. In addition, virtue in Western medicine includes an explicit commitment to scientific truth itself, founded on the deeply held conviction that medical knowledge is a precious and hard-won gemstone, wrested from the bedrock of ignorance by dint of great effort. This commitment to truth, and the scientific method that generates knowledge, constitute one of the core medical values that will preserve our identity as physicians as long as we honor it.

The Biopsychosocial Model

A second pillar of psychiatry's medical identity is the biopsychosocial model (Engel 1977). The biopsychosocial model can be understood as an extension of the medical model to the realm of behavior in an attempt to connect the primary medical locus of our work, namely the brain and its pathology, with the experience of mind, on the one hand, and with interpersonal/social systems, on the other. Here our field demonstrates both its unique strengths and contributions to medicine and its vulnerability to ridicule. By conceptualizing human behavior simultaneously on multiple, different levels and making interventions with the family, with the medication, with the employer, and with the psyche, the field appears at times diffuse, nonspecific, even self-contradictory. This is because the biopsychosocial model intentionally allows for, even demands, tremendous diversity of explanation. It also relies on an open systems perspective as opposed to a closed, linear perspective. And it is just at this point that critics can claim the field is "soft" and take advantage of real ambiguity and clinical uncertainty to challenge the very therapeutic enterprise itself, as when the reviewer just wants to raise the dose of the neuroleptic of a slow-to-respond patient and does not want to hear about family issues, ambivalence, or anxiety due to deficient social skills (Sharfstein 1992). Clearly the field will not abandon its understanding of the importance of these hard-to-quantify domains and their interactions. If, however, it deals with managed care simply by ceasing to talk about them to reviewers, it risks reinforcing the managed care perception that they are not "real" in the first place.

The Hippocratic Model of the Doctor-Patient Relationship

The third leg upon which psychiatry stands as a medical specialty is the Hippocratic model of the doctor-patient relationship. By virtue of its medical identity, psychiatry shares the 2,400-year-old legacy of personal responsibility and commitment to the individual patient that characterizes the soul of Western medicine. Psychiatry is the only member of the larger team of mental health disciplines that has this Hippocratic heritage. Psychiatrists alone among mental health providers have carried the life and death burden of decision making about dying patients and have gone through the purgatory of being "on call." The importance of this experience, specifically as it bears on the internalization of the Hippocratic value system, can hardly be overstated.

The significance of the doctor-patient relationship for psychiatry, born of this travail, is in turn not to be minimized. This deeply emotional bond accounts for the tremendous sacrifices doctors have historically made for their patients (more evident, to be sure in the era before health insurance, but still ongoing). Likewise, the terrible sense of ethical wrongdoing experienced by many doctors as they face choices imposed on them by today's managed care stems from what is instinctively felt as a violation of the prohibition to "do no harm." Finally, Hippocratic tradition is the foundation of our identity as a profession, as opposed to being merely employees.

The American Medical Association's and the American Psychiatric Association's Principles of Ethics are derived from Percival's code. They include a statement of our obligation not only to the patient (per the Hippocratic model) but also to self and society. The physician's obligation to society is murky and causes difficulty in interpretation especially when in conflict with other commitments. In the absence of clarification, however, the patient advocacy role must take preeminence.

The Hippocratic model has also provided the *legal* definition for physician responsibility in the United States. The present status of tort law in America clearly assumes a traditional Hippocratic relationship as the basis for the physician's personal liability for malpractice. Although not suggesting that the present state of malpractice litigation in the United States is a good thing, we do point out that a major impetus for quality and responsibility in health care is expressed in this legal embodiment of the Hippocratic doctor-patient relationship.

Taken together, this triad of medical, biopsychosocial, and Hippocratic models forms an impressive footing upon which to build an identity. Its interdependent components strengthen one another and generate a coherent whole that is more than the sum of its parts.

Managed Care

Medicine as Product

Let us turn then for a moment to examine the ways in which the practice of psychiatry is currently being challenged. Panzetta (Schreter, Sharfstein, and Schreter 1994) has articulated an admittedly overdrawn exposition of the current managed care view of psychiatry. Managed care, first of all, must be clearly defined as a business enterprise. It is a quintessential expression of American capitalism. From the perspective of business, medicine and psychiatry are mere components in a specific case of production and consumption, no different from any other. Psychiatrists become, in such a model, expensive labor whose utilization must be rationalized. The principles driving the rationalization of labor, however, are far different from what we have just discussed. Business is not interested in the intrinsic value of the medical, biopsychosocial, or Hippocratic models. The marketplace is value neutral. Business has passing interest in values only insofar as they relate to the competitiveness of its product. And if its product can be sold without having to pay for the costs associated with values, it will try to do so unless constrained by external forces. This is one reason why government exists.

Hence, in managed care, the rationalization of psychiatric labor leads to the recurrent theme, "What aspects of psychiatric care can be done more cheaply by less expensive labor?" This is a far cry from a medically based rationalization, which would start with the question, "What serves the interest of the patient best, and how can the psychiatrist, drawing upon the medical, biopsychosocial, and Hippocratic models, contribute most effectively and efficiently toward that end?" The managed care perspective can lead to a fragmentation of the psychiatrist's identity. Because cheaper labor is perceived as able to create equivalent products in several domains of psychiatry, such as psychotherapy, the managed care provider simply mandates such amputations by fiat, cutting psychiatry back to those sole activities of production that are clearly reserved to physicians by virtue of medical training or law. Moreover, even those domains clearly associated with medicine are further constricted and mangled as the standard of quality becomes defined by customer satisfaction, market share, and profit margin rather than medical values. At its worst, the creature that emerges from such surgery is a pale shadow of its former self: the psychiatrist as pill pusher, form signer, hassle fixer, crisis manager, and worst of all, denier of needed care.

Outcome Studies

Now the managed care apologist may respond that this caricature is unfair and that, although some abuses in quality of care may indeed have occurred thus far in the evolution of the business, this is merely a "transitional" or "start-up" problem that will be resolved in the next iteration of the "product." To bolster this claim, we hear about "outcome studies," which managed care tells us will "add value" to their "quality product." But is this really so? Unfortunately, studies published so far have been essentially marketing surveys. Up to now, the best minds in the research community, who have wrestled with the measurement of outcomes for the past 30 years, have not been recruited by managed care to lead the effort in collecting scientifically valid data from which honest conclusions can be drawn. In fact, we would assert that any measurement of outcomes must by definition assume familiarity with the medical, biopsychosocial, and Hippocratic models. We focus on this issue of outcome research because we believe it highlights an essential difference between medicine and business. To reiterate, the medical model is based on science and virtue. It has an inherent commitment to distinguish what is true from what is false, in this instance what constitutes a truly beneficial outcome and not just a satisfied consumer, however important that, too, may be. Physicians are custodians of an accumulated mass of medical knowledge that is true, at least for the moment, until better knowledge is generated. And no matter how tenuous such distinctions are at times of great ignorance, it is this fundamental commitment to truth that drives, empowers, and ennobles the whole enterprise.

Where does this leave us, then? We must return to the driving force behind these events: a very real scarcity of resources in a time of increased needs. How can psychiatry address this problem proactively while maintaining a secure hold on its core values?

The Clinical Essentials of Quality Psychiatric Care

We would like to turn now to a more detailed examination of the components and processes involved in the praxis of psychiatric medicine, particularly as it pertains to the impact on it by scarce resources. The requirements are really relatively few and straightforward. You must start with a foundation of correct diagnosis and formulation of the case. You must then select the correct treatment(s) and either implement them yourself or delegate them. You must subsequently ensure that multiple treatment interventions are coordinated and assess the efficacy of your interventions. And finally, somewhere in all of this, there usually needs to be a sustaining relationship with the patient, either explicitly in one of the treatments or implicitly in the overall system as it is set up.

Information

Now, what does the therapeutic context need to provide the psychiatrist in order for to this to happen? First of all, the psychiatrist needs *information*. The psychiatric specialty oral boards explicitly assess candidates on their ability to rapidly glean, organize, differentiate, integrate, remember, evaluate, and judge clinical information. Next to integrity and logic, that is what academic medicine values most highly. And this is as it should be by whatever standard one uses, be it psychoanalytic, biological, phenomenological, or cognitive/behavioral. All the prevailing therapeutic models are complex, sophisticated, multivariate open systems that require *data* to produce meaningful results. Moreover, nowadays we often contemplate the parallel and/or interactive effects of two or more such models *simultaneously*. That is part of the intellectual excitement in psychiatry! But to train doctors in such complex heuristic models and then deny them the data to properly implement the model, yet still maintain to the public that they are receiving quality care because, after all, a doctor is "doing it," promulgates only an illusion of expertise that does not bear close scrutiny of what "it" is. This is nonetheless exactly what happens whenever managed care reviewers intentionally, or public-sector poverty unintentionally, force psychiatrists to make too rapid assessments and dispositions without the benefit of data. But beware! The lack of information collected about patients does not mean that the problems and considerations we have been trained to look for and understand do not exist. The absence of a written history does not mean the patient does not have a history.

Time

In order to collect, synthesize, and act intelligently upon the information so carefully gathered, the psychiatrist also needs time. Time is a critical element in psychiatric assessment and treatment because, although there may be time without information (i.e., the old psychoanalytic free-association days), there is never information without time. Time is also needed for the dynamic aspects of a case to be understood because the systems under scrutiny are not stable, but in flux. Single point in time, cross-sectional, evaluations are, as good clinicians know all too well, fraught with hazards.

Of course, the managed care provider, ever the good businessperson, knows that "time is money." And so we have already seen in recent years the savaging of time allocated to patient care. The clinical consequences of this are very real. The irrational and arbitrary constriction of clinical time is wreaking havoc on many of our patients' treatments. At our institution, for example, we have children coming from tremendously disturbed environments, with horrendous, complex, and manifold problems, whose inpatient treatment costs society thousands and thousands of dollars. In this inpatient setting, however, a psychiatrist actually has *less* time during the first week with the patient than almost any private outpatient psychiatrist would have, who would charge a few hundred dollars to do a comprehensive consultation over the course of two or three office visits! The obsession with cost, which escalates to a near frenzy with any inpatient stay, actually undoes much of the value of the hospitalization in the first place. It therefore is a self-fulfilling prophecy to pronounce, "Hospitalization is only good for safety containment anyway." Obviously, it is if you eliminate some of its key ingredients.

Time is equally necessary for the implementation and coordination of treatment. We are not talking here about intensive psychotherapy. We mean that the practice of psychiatry, using any modality, requires the constant collection of yet ever new data (e.g., the reassessment of mental status, the updating of recent personal events, the evaluation of emotional reactions and behavior, and so on), and this simply cannot be done in 15 minutes when a patient is the slightest bit unstable or even just undergoing expected change.

Finally, time is necessary for the cultivation of any relationship. Of course, if the agenda is to save money by saving time, then the systematic undermining of any opportunity to establish human relationships may be exactly what is intended.

The Psychiatrist Defined

What special qualities, skills, and perspectives does the psychiatrist bring to the mental health team?

The Whole Patient

A further word about the significance of the biopsychosocial model is called for here. This model is an expression of concern for the "whole patient." As the rest of medicine has hurdled headlong into ever increasing subspecialization during the past 30 years, the biopsychosocial model has allowed psychiatry to maintain a perspective on the person, even as it, too, has become fascinated with receptors and genes instead of people. It is perhaps because psychiatry continues ultimately to deal with people as psyche, and not just as receptors, that we have maintained this perspective. It is quite ironic, in fact, that just as society, in the voice of the President himself, clamors for less subspecialization and a return to care of the whole patient, that psychiatry, a historic spokesperson for this value, is in danger of itself becoming a neurological subspecialty.

The psychiatrist's training puts him or her in a position to view, in depth, the entire range of potential influences that may bear upon a clinical situation. Moreover, the biopsychosocial model, as a systems perspective, encourages a wide-ranging inquiry into the breadth of possible influences and into their manifest (and sometimes covert) *interactions* as well. It downplays the narrow focus on a single symptom and instead asks, "What are the hidden forces that contribute to the apparent problem (e.g., the chief complaint) as presented by the patient, family, or others?" This perspective is not mere window dressing. Tremendous wastage and inefficiencies, even outright bad patient care, result at this very moment because a narrow perspective dictates practice. Consider the following example:

> A 24-year-old woman with depression is treated with bupropion. On a hike in a rural park with her boyfriend, she experiences a seizure. He does not witness this but does find her groggy on the rocks. Because of her facial lacerations, he assumes she has slipped and fallen and

sustained a head injury. Other hikers go for help, and soon the medevac helicopter arrives and whisks her off to the shock trauma center at the major metropolitan teaching hospital. There, skilled surgeons assess her for closed head injury, using state-of-the-art imaging machines. The lacerations are stitched, and the patient is discharged. No one asks about the bupropion or the patient's depression, no one calls the patient's psychiatrist (who is available by beeper), no one does an EEG, no one does a tox screen or gets a blood level. So, after all this expense and sophisticated trauma care, the patient goes out and has another seizure 24 hours later.

This example is not meant to laud or fault any one specialty. Psychiatrists could just as well have ignored the potential consequences of medical or surgical treatments: The "usual" somatic complaints of a therapy patient are "interpreted," whereas appendicitis goes undetected; the bradykinesia and dulling in a patient early in the course of Parkinson's disease are written off as depression. One hopes that the medical training of a contemporary psychiatrist is exactly what will make such an event *unlikely!* We simply want to emphasize how *any* overly narrow focus, shaped in some ways by the very questions that a strong explanatory model or a powerful technology are designed to address, can lead to erroneous diagnoses and poor or inappropriate medical care. A broader systems perspective, which includes knowledge of the patient as a whole, can be a powerful antidote to such distortions.

The skeptic may still retort that such oversights are going to happen occasionally. Is it really cost effective to build in safeguards against such "rare events"? For after all, what we are suggesting requires yet more resources. In this particular case, for example, one might consider having a consultation/liaison psychiatrist consult on any trauma case of a psychiatric patient or having a clinician routinely call any outpatient doctors involved in a case. A cost-conscious administrator might point to outcome data that would purport to "prove" that such greater staffing yields no statistically significant difference in morbidity/mortality. But we ask you, what model of outcome analysis will be sophisticated enough to address this sort of event? And how do we weigh the real human cost to the individual who has the second seizure? We are not saying that such an analysis could never be done. But we do wonder if it would ever be economically and logistically feasible, given how many variables and interacting systems would need to be accounted for. There are outcomes and complications that can be readily understood by clinicians, but not so readily modeled. Must we then ignore them just because we cannot model them? Does it mean they do not exist?

Training

This broad perspective is obviously a direct outcome of the psychiatrist's training, which is unique among the mental health team. As doctors, psychiatrists are the result of *a social screening process* that begins in college and continues for 12 years of training. Such screening selects for certain characteristics, including intelligence, perseverance, and ethical integrity. The fact that some doctors make the headlines as notoriously lacking one or more of these characteristics does not, in our opinion, detract from the intrinsic value of this winnowing process in principle (though it does raise important questions about the ability of the medical profession to enforce its own standards at times!) Included in this 12-year educational process is explicit training in, and expectation of, team leadership. Psychiatrists receive more hours of instruction and clinical supervision than any other mental health discipline. They receive specialized training in the treatment of the more seriously ill spectrum of patients. They are the legally identified team members with authority to admit to hospitals in most states and countries, as well as to certify patients involuntarily, order restraints, and authorize a wide variety of social and treatment interventions such as disability claims, referrals to expensive treatment programs, and so on. Psychiatrists are also best suited to interacting with the other medical/surgical physicians on the patient's case as a peer and colleague.

Research

A tremendously important contribution of the psychiatrist is research. The psychiatrist carries out society's commitment to understanding the etiology, pathogenesis, and treatment of major mental illness. The psychiatrist is again the only mental health team member whose training, at least theoretically, enables him or her to interact with biochemists, geneticists, neurophysiologists, epidemiologists, and so on as a medically conversant and competent peer. Of course, there are highly gifted and well-trained psychologists who operate at this level, too, but as a discipline, psychiatry *systematically* produces a group of researchers perfectly primed to enter into this kind of biomedical research.

Payment

Finally, lest we be accused of dodging the tough issues, we must acknowledge that psychiatrists are the most highly paid members of the mental health team. This is no small point and in some ways might be considered the first item for discussion, not the last. For after all, were this not true, would we even be having this debate? Whatever comes of national health reform, however, it is probable that psychiatrists will continue to be the most highly paid members of the mental health team. Whether the disparity between reimbursement to psychiatrists and the other mental health disciplines stays as great as it is currently remains to be seen. One could argue in fact that far from paying psychiatrists less, society should be paying nonmedical psychotherapists more (and demanding in return better training and certification requirements to boot)! Whether sufficient resources exist for this is uncertain, but, in any event, it seems highly unlikely in our society that professionals with extensive training, expertise, and responsibility will not be rewarded proportionally.

The Role of the Psychiatrist in a New Era

Having characterized what the psychiatrist ideally brings to the treatment team caring for psychiatric patients, let us now consider how psychiatric expertise and talent can be most effectively used as an expensive and scarce resource.

Diagnosis will always be an inherent role of the psychiatrist, even as an implicit confirmatory second opinion. For example, the physician will not prescribe medications for a patient referred to him or her as "depressed" by a nonphysician without agreeing on the diagnosis.

Medication management, that deceptively simple catchphrase we have been hearing so much of lately, is another psychiatric role even in routine cases. The process of medicating patients in collaboration with the psychotherapist and/or other mental health care providers is not as simple as merely writing out a few prescriptions. If sufficient information is not obtained from the patient and/or the collaborating team members, the psychiatrist will be left in the dark as to what is really going on with a patient. Such information requires a minimal amount of contact with the collaborators, as well as sufficient rapport with the patient so that the patient will verbalize key information in a relatively brief time. Medication management can become a difficult and delicate juggling act if disagreements arise between the psychiatrist and the therapist. Conflicts arising from differences in perspective, training, or philosophy can in complex cases lead to ethical dilemmas: When should one advise the patient that one disagrees with the therapist? When should one disengage from a case that is being mishandled? Psychiatrists must also be alert to the legal complexities in the medication management role. Sufficient time with the patient is necessary if one is to anticipate and avoid potential malpractice actions against the psychiatrist, who may still be considered ultimately accountable in the current legal environment, even if his or her contact with the patient is minimal.

The role of *consultant* also enables psychiatrists to be used efficiently. Here, a discrete problem is encountered by one or more members of the treatment team, and the psychiatrist is involved not necessarily for his or her biomedical expertise but for his or her broader background, education, experience, and, on occasion, objectivity. As primary care physicians are directed to take over more and more initial treatment of simple psychiatric disorders, the psychiatrist consultant also will likely have an important role in capitated systems, especially those with psychiatric carve outs that lack their own psychiatric staff.

Historically, *team leadership* has been another integral role of the psychiatrist. In recent years this, too, has eroded in some settings, again largely for economic reasons. However, we are now seeing sicker and sicker patients being treated outside of the hospital, and as managed care moves to assume responsibility for the public sector, the deliberate and carefully considered adaptation of the inpatient team model to new settings presents an exciting new clinical opportunity for psychiatrists to assume a leadership role. We would argue that if outpatient multidisciplinary services are going to be delivered well, a coherent team is crucial to effective service, and that a psychiatrist should be explicitly identified *and empowered* to play the role of team leader in appropriate cases. In future vertically integrated systems of psychiatric care, the concept of comprehensive team leadership will probably also include supervision of treatment planning, educational activities directed toward inexperienced and less well trained members of the team, and overall utilization review. This comprehensive role will likely be directly influenced by data acquired through continuous quality improvement outcomes databases, and the psychiatrist/team leader will be a critical linchpin in "closing the loop" between service delivery and efficacy of the treatment system. The justification for making the psychiatrist such a comprehensive team leader is straightforward enough: It is founded on the amount of training, the breadth of perspective needed to ensure the highest quality care, and the ultimate accountability of the doctor. The typical day of such a team leader will likely be quite different from traditional psychotherapeutic office practice, but it offers the potential for genuine satisfaction and an opportunity to make a unique contribution to quality patient care, for those so inclined.

Finally, the psychiatrist is still likely to provide direct, total psychiatric care in the *integrated treatment of patients in complex cases*. By complex we mean cases where the patient's pathology is so severe and dangerous, so organic, so fluid and pleomorphic, or so exploitative of the psychiatrist/team split that the patient and treatment team both suffer by trying to fragment and limit the psychiatrist's role. Such cases might involve the following:

- Unstable psychotic or mood disordered or organic patients with rapidly changing phenomenology and need for medication changes
- Severe characterological/dissociative patients with demonstrated manipulative splitting
- Seriously medically ill patients
- Seriously suicidal patients
- Seriously substance abusing patients

- Atypical patients who are out of the experience range of other team members
- Highly dangerous forensic cases
- Cases where litigious or manipulative families or patients unilaterally insist that they "want" a doctor as therapist

The following is an example:

> RJ was a 27-year-old male with schizoaffective disorder who had a history of several hospitalizations for psychosis and suicidal behavior. In our continuum of care, he was residing in a highly structured group home with 24-hour supervision and using a specialized inpatient unit for hospitalization when it was necessary. He had an outpatient psychiatrist for medications, different inpatient psychiatrists each time he was hospitalized, and a day hospital. At first there was no therapy. After the second hospitalization, a Ph.D. psychologist was assigned as a therapist, and the patient was assigned to yet another psychiatrist for medication management. He was quite unstable and was hospitalized two more times. The outpatient medicating psychiatrist found it very difficult to get a handle on the case, even with weekly medication visits and frequent discussions with the psychologist and housing and day hospital staff (none of which calls were allowed for in the psychiatrist's "productivity" assessment, by the way). The psychiatrist finally asked to become the patient's therapist and began to see the patient weekly for 50-minute therapy sessions. The patient was very verbal and opened up to the psychiatrist, revealing a great deal of informative delusional and historical material that had direct bearing on his unstable behavior. The patient settled down, the diagnostic considerations became clear (after two years of uncertainty), and not only was the patient not rehospitalized in the following 15 months, but he was successfully discharged to a supervised apartment in the community.

This case illustrates a situation where more was less: where the proliferation of a fragmented team, to none of whose members the patient was really attached, led to the psychiatric equivalent of "the lab work was all normal but the patient expired!" Here, we were doing "all the right things" by the current book of multidisciplinary, cost-effective use of resources, but the patient was not doing well.

The decision to combine the therapist and psychiatrist function was paid for by the patient's indemnity insurance; it would have resulted in an increase in cost to a capitated system. But the net payoff for a capitated system or for an indemnity insurer exposed to long-term risk was substantial: Hospitalization was reduced, and the patient moved to progressively less costly residential options.

In summary, it is our view that there are limits to the effectiveness of psychiatrists as consultants or medicators, and those limits are defined by the very nature and complexity of our work. Of course, it is possible to conceive the task narrowly and *go through the motions* of delivering psychiatric care "from afar." In fact, it is easier (so long as one does not have a conscience) because if the patient does poorly, there is less personal responsibility. It becomes the patient's fault, usually, and the system just keeps grinding along, readmitting the patient and spitting him or her out again, as in the revolving-door syndrome seen in many deinstitutionalized patients. This is particularly likely to happen in fee-for-service models that lack a continuum of care. If funded adequately (a big if), capitated models, we believe, hold the promise of surmounting this kind of superficial psychiatry and addressing the systems problems that confront the whole patient, and not just the inpatient or the outpatient. For this to work, however, the psychiatrist's role will have to be conceptualized flexibly—as flexibly as we have always prided ourselves on conceptualizing the patient.

Controversial Visions of the Future Psychiatrist

The Psychiatrist Who Does No Psychotherapy

Much has already been said over the past decade about the role of psychotherapy training and practice for the modern psychiatrist (Verhuist 1991). Some feel that "medical psychotherapy" is an outdated holdover from another era, an anachronism in effect. A recent editorial in the *Lancet* (1994) recommended a bifurcation of the field to formalize a division that it contends has already occurred. It should be clear from the preceding remarks that we do not share this view.

The psychotherapeutic heritage that our profession shares speaks to the very heart of the biopsychosocial model and is absolutely essential to the functioning of psychiatry as we have just described it. It is obviously a prerequisite for the psychiatrist to be able to handle complex cases independently, and it follows that the skills to handle such cases are greater than those sufficient to provide treatment in routine ones. Likewise, one cannot expect a psychiatrist to supervise other mental health professionals who are doing psychotherapy without expertise in the activity he or she is supervising. No mere "exposure" to psychotherapy as an "elective" will suffice in such situations. If psychotherapeutically untrained psychiatrists do attempt to assert team leadership even in the absence of genuine skills, they risk being held in secret contempt by the other disciplines. Team members will consult with the psychiatrist "just" for medication-related issues, medical questions, or legal hassles that they want to avoid, while reserving the real psychological core of the case to themselves because they do not respect the psychiatrist's psychotherapeutic wisdom and even see him or her as less well trained and sensitive than they are. This is already happening in some settings. Such animosity and disrespect surely do not bode well for a sound collegial and cooperative approach to patient care.

Even beyond treatment in complex cases, however, the psychiatrist needs to maintain some amount of psychotherapeutic activity *for the proper functioning of all the other roles*. This is because psychotherapy is the only way to maintain an appreciation of the complexity of the biopsychosocial model and not allow oneself to become deluded by overly simplistic, reductionistic explanations of behavior, such as the oft repeated assertion by staff, "the patient just needs more meds." People are more complicated than that. Psychotherapeutic skills also improve the ability of the neuropsychiatrist to function on his or her own turf by enabling interviewing skills that produce more information directly pertinent to the understanding of both the biology and context of the illness. A checklist approach to interviewing, although helpful in guaranteeing thoroughness, can lead to inaccurate information if used insensitively, with the result being, "garbage in, garbage out."

Psychotherapy also protects against countertransference distortions because its very perspective invites and requires a continual review of countertransference experiences. No amount of neuropsychiatric superstructure is going to change the reality that psychiatric patients affect the people around them viscerally and powerfully. Even if buffered from the emotional heat of the patient by the rest of the team, the neuropsychiatrist will miss the essentials of a case if he or she is unable to include this intersubjectivity as a part of the overall formulation of what is going on. The neuropsychiatrist will remain part of the patient's interpersonal system, whether his or her perspective has room for this or not, and it is incumbent on the neuropsychiatrist to be self-aware and responsive to such forces.

On the other hand, if one concedes in principle the value of the psychotherapeutic endeavor for the identity of the practicing psychiatrist, there is still the option to limit its place in the overall time distribution of the psychiatrist's daily activities. How much, in effect, is enough? This will vary from person to person, but it seems to us that 10% of a psychiatrist's time is a bare minimum to be spent doing psychotherapy in order to maintain essential skills, with 20%–25% being preferable lest that 10% be just "the impossible cases" that drain the psychiatrist. Burnout is a real concern for a revised role of the psychiatrist, and maintaining a minimum psychotherapy experience with a few treatment-responsive patients is an effective antidote to that eventuality.

The Psychiatrist as "Principal Physician"

In another view of the future, the psychiatrist becomes the principal medical physician for a significant portion of his or her caseload, providing primary medical care for coexisting Axis III diagnoses such as uncomplicated hypertension, congestive heart failure, diabetes, infections, and so on. Such a concept could further bolster psychiatry's identity as a branch of mainstream medicine and contribute to society's perceived need for more primary care providers. The actual intermingling of psychiatrists with other physicians, necessitated by equal access to medically equipped office space, would address a major physical gulf that literally separates most psychiatrists from their medical colleagues at present. Such a model would be particularly well suited to certain groups of psychiatric patients who traditionally have not received good medical care from conventional delivery systems. These would include the chronically mentally ill, highly somaticizing patients, and disturbed borderline patients who act out around their medical illnesses. The consolidation of the principal physician's role with that of the psychiatrist could do much to address the fragmentation of medical care these patients often experience. It could perhaps even reduce the resources currently being wasted when specialists who do not know them and their context order unnecessary tests and treatments.

There are major problems with implementing such a model, however. To begin with, it would require significant changes in training, with at least one more year of medical residency needed. The cost of upgrading office space to provide lab access, examination rooms, not to mention support staff salaries for nurses, would be considerable. It would be critically important that the resources directed to such remodeling be truly equivalent to other sites of primary care, to preclude the principal physician-psychiatrist being viewed as a "not quite" doctor delivering a lower level of care, an eventuality that the cultural countertransference to these patient populations might well encourage in subtle ways. From the psychiatric point of view, such remodeling would present a significantly increased burden of maintaining competency in two domains of expertise. The explosion of information to be kept up within both psychiatry and medicine would require careful attention to ensure that sufficient opportunity for study be built in, lest the level of care be allowed to drift down to the lowest common denominator instead of being pushed toward the state of the art.

Conclusion

American psychiatry today is at a critical historical juncture. It has reached a pinnacle of success in terms of developing treatments for mental illness, generating new data about the etiology and pathogenesis of neuropsychiatric disorders, and, perhaps most important, establishing an intellectually rigorous research *method* that has laid the groundwork for an entire generation of psychiatrists to carry this progress still further. At stake when we talk about the evolution of the psychiatrist's identity is the future success of this extremely productive intellectual endeavor that may be mortally jeopardized in the name of economy and equity. The redistribution and rationalization of resources are, to be sure, an inherent good: We genuinely embrace and endorse this commitment to the common good. But the field must at the same time protect its core identity, lest those very forces that *allow* for much needed social change unwittingly *distort and corrupt* the very services they are trying to make more generally available in the first place.

To prevent this, psychiatry must proactively assert what we think we should become in the overall system of reformed health care in America and then see to it that we do what needs to be done in the interim to ensure that we get there. Toward that end, we make one very specific recommendation, beyond the more general values espoused in this chapter. We concur with Yager and Borus (Borus and Yager 1986; Yager and Borus 1987) that *American psychiatry has settled for standards that are too low.* By allowing for great professional diversity and even encouraging such in the name of creativity and intellectual humility, the profession has come to permit some of our members to be unqualified for what society expects of us. There is excessive variance in our practice, some of it frankly bad, and a good deal of it unsupported by scientific evidence. In this respect, good managed care is delivering a needed wake-up call to the profession in the guise of mandated peer review, which has been sorely lacking in all of medicine, including psychiatry, sad to say. In our opinion, in other words, there is merit in managed care's assertion that much of what they deny is indeed inferior or unjustifiable psychiatric care.

One place to redress this problem proactively is the board qualification and certification process. We need to review the entire curriculum and the standards for graduation from training programs, which currently graduate 96% of their candidates. There needs to be a vigorous collaboration among the American Association of Directors of Residency Training, the Accreditation Council for Graduate Medical Education, the American Board of Psychiatry and Neurology, *and* the clinical leadership of the managed care industry. Such an effort should be directed toward identifying standards of practice based on the available research literature and a consensus of clinical experts. There should be much greater emphasis on teaching the development of specific treatment plans, where the demands of limited resources, medical research, and real patient needs meet.

Psychiatry residency programs should upgrade their academic expectations of residents, perhaps by systematically using the fourth year (often a kind of throwaway year) in a more scholarly way. We support the model of the *clinician scientist:* that is, the physician who is versed in the most current research literature, whose clinical decisions are based on that literature when it is available, and whose allegiance is to the quest for scientific evidence above any ideology or nonscientific epistemology. This already is the model in internal medicine and its subspecialties. For example, the internal medicine boards publish a list of research studies for which the candidate will be held accountable on the exam. Psychiatry could easily do the same: The literature is there! We are riding the crest of a research wave and should make mastery of this knowledge the expectation of the credentialed specialist and not just the purview of scholars.

Here are examples of some of the things we *could* do: 1) make board certification a requirement for reimbursement three years after graduation from residency, 2) mandate universal recertification (eliminating the current hypocritical grandfathered loophole), and 3) increase the difficulty level of the boards with a heavy emphasis on research-justified treatment planning. Such actions would take much of the clout from managed care by ensuring that psychiatrists had mastered the knowledge base to practice the highest quality psychiatry in the first place. The profession could then face the criticisms leveled at it by medicine, by third parties, and by other mental health disciplines from a position of *proven* competency and expertise. Now is the time: The knowledge base finally exists! If such a transformation decreased the number of psychiatrists, thus forcing the psychiatrist as consultant model to be even more likely an outcome, so be it: At least the consultant would be a real expert. In our view, such a transformation toward higher standards would have the opposite effect, however. By ensuring that only competent and well-trained physicians are credentialed as psychiatrists, we would increase the credibility of the field as a whole, thus enticing medical students to join a profession with a commitment to both patient care and intellectual excellence. Such an outcome could only strengthen the identity of a renewed and generative profession.

References

Borus J, Yager J: Ongoing evaluation in psychiatry: the first step toward quality. Am J Psychiatry 143: 1415–1419, 1986
Dyer AR: Ethics and Psychiatry: Toward Professional Definition. Washington, DC, American Psychiatric Press, 1988
Editorial: Molecules and minds. Lancet 343.8899:681–682, 1994
Engel G: The need for a new medical model: a challenge for biomedicine. Science 196:129, 1977
Schreter RK, Sharfstein SS, Schreter CA (eds): Allies and Adversaries: The Impact of Managed Care on Mental Health Services. Washington, DC, American Psychiatric Press, 1994
Sharfstein SS: Managed Mental Health Care. American Psychiatric Association Annual Update. Edited by Gabbard G, Munich R. Washington, DC, American Psychiatric Press, 1992
Verhuist J: The psychotherapy curriculum in the age of biological psychiatry: mixing oil with water? Academic Psychiatry 15:120–131, 1991
Yager J, Borus J: Are we training too many psychiatrists? Am J Psychiatry 144:1042–1048, 1987

Index

Academic psychiatry, collaboration with managed behavioral health care
 barriers to, 112–115
 objectives for, 115–119
 overview, 111–112
 suggestions for, 119–121
 See also Psychiatry departments
Administrative psychiatry, 76–79. *See also* Managed behavioral health care
Ambulatory care, in new medical marketplace, 16–17
American Association of Chairmen of Departments of Psychiatry, 113
American Association of Directors of Psychiatric Residency Training, 113
American Hospital Association, 216
American Medical Association (AMA)
 "Breaking the Capitation Bronco," 176
 ethics principles, 147, 191–192
 See also Council on Ethical and Judicial Affairs
American Psychiatric Association (APA), practice guidelines of, 193

Americans with Disabilities Act (ADA), and ERISA-based discrimination, 201–202
Ancillary risk, 171
Antitrust laws, 191, 206–207
Any willing provider (AWP) laws, 220–221
Asylums. *See* Public mental health sites
Autonomy model, for physician-patient relationship, 142–143

Behavioral health care, industrialization of, 131–133. *See also* Managed behavioral health care
Biomedical care, psychiatric responsibilities in, 47, 240–242
Biopsychosocial model, 240–241, 247
Blue Cross & Blue Shield, 212–213, 215–216
Bonus incentives, 171, 175
"Breaking the Capitation Bronco" (AMA), 176

Califano, Joseph, 213
Capitation, 171
 effects of, 221–224
 ethical issues, 176, 178
 HMO as example of, 224–228

261

Capitation *(continued)*
for psychiatric services, 175
with risk-sharing mechanisms, 173
Carve ins, 229–231
Carve outs, 224–228
Certificates of need (CON) requirements, 149
Clinical administration, role of psychiatrists in, 48
Clinician scientist, model of, 259
Clinton Administration
and Consumer Bill of Rights and Responsibilities, 100
health care reform plan, 15, 34, 97, 197
Command and control regulation, 190–191, 197
Community Mental Health Center (CMHC) Act, 6–7
Community-wide hospital plans, 216–217
Competition, as challenge for psychiatrists, 50–51
Comprehensive reform, 14–15
Computerized databases, as UR tool, 219–220
Confidentiality, 91
and managed care, 161–165
in physician-patient relationship, 147–148
See also Ethical issues; Privacy
Consultants, psychiatrists' role as, 251
Consultation
outpatient, with PCPs, 65–66
psychiatric, 47–48

Consumer Bill of Rights and Responsibilities, 100
Consumer demand, for quality care, 25
Continuity, in psychiatrist-patient relationship, 91–92
Continuous quality improvement (CQI), 30
Cost control strategies, 10–15. *See also* Managed care
Council on Ethical and Judicial Affairs (CEJA), draft report recommendations
clinical practice guidelines, 152–153
financial incentives, 154, 157–158
informed consent, 161
patient advocacy and participation, 153
summary, 141–142
County mental hospitals. *See* Public mental health sites
Crisis assessment, 60

Data, and quality care, 245. *See also* Outcomes data
Databases, computerized, as UR tool, 219–220
Demand-side cost control methods, 10–11
Diagnosis, 250
Diagnosis related groups (DRGs), 149–150, 221–222
Disclosure. *See* Informed consent
Discount pricing. *See* Negotiated discounts

Index

Disincentives, 169–170
    ethical issues, 176–178
    in medicine, 170–174
    in psychiatry, 174–176
    suggested solutions for, 178–181
Doctor-patient relationship. *See* Physician-patient relationship
Duke University, Department of Psychiatry, 113

"Economic informed consent," 176–177
Economic reforms, in 1970s, 7–15
Employment Retirement Income Security Act (ERISA), 190, 196–202
Ethical issues
    for determining quality care, 26–29
    for financial incentives, 173–174, 176–178
    in new medical marketplace, 21
    See also Confidentiality; Moral paradigm; Physician-patient relationship; Privacy

Federal Trade Commission (FTC), and AMA's ethics principles, 192, 193
Fee-for-service (FFS) reimbursement, 8, 12
    effect on physician-patient relationship, 151
    in private practice, 98–99
    utilization review of, 210–213
    See also Financial incentives
Financial incentives, 169–170
    conflicts between physicians and patients, 154–158
    ethical issues, 176–178
    in medicine, 170–174
    for private practitioners, 95
    in psychiatry, 174–176
    suggested solutions for, 178–181
    See also Capitation; Fee-for-service (FFS) reimbursement
"Fiscal informed consent," 159
Fourth-party utilization review, 210–213
Funding, for psychiatric training, 119

Gatekeeping, 152, 172–173, 230
Government, role in promoting quality care, 33–35
Government regulations
    antitrust laws, 191, 206–207
    AWP laws, 220–221
    of health services, 25–26
    limiting provider control, 213
    vs. market solutions, 190–193
    for referrals, 207
    See also Employment Retirement Income Security Act (ERISA)
Guidelines. *See* Practice guidelines

Harvard Community Health Plan, 113, 117
Harvard Longwood Psychiatry Training Program, 113
Health care, quality of. *See* Quality care
"Health care cost crisis," 7–15
Health Care Finance Administration (HCFA), UR committees, 149
Health care reform, 3–4
  economic reforms in 1970s, 7–15
  emergence of medical marketplace, 15–21
  and market forces, 72–73
  social reforms in 1960s, 4–7
  See also Clinton Administration, health care reform plan
Health Maintenance Organizations (HMOs)
  as example of capitation system, 224–228
  for-profit shift in, 208
  Harvard Community Health Plan, 113, 117
  outcomes data on, 98–99
  public backlash against, 99–100
  recruitment of Medicare patients, 195
  structure of, 150
  See also Managed behavioral health care; Managed care
Health Plan Employer Data and Information Set (HEDIS 3.0), 33

Health services, quality in. *See* Quality care
High-risk patients, management of, 60–61
Hippocratic model, of doctor-patient relationship, 241–242
HMO Act of 1973, 10, 170
Horizontal integration, 209, 231. *See also* Selective contracting
Hospitals
  community-wide plans, 216–217
  downsizing of, 15–16
  and DRGs, 221–222
  as "health systems," 17
  and oligopsony purchasing power, 205–206
Human economies of scale, 223, 226, 227–228, 230

Iglehart, John, 196–197
Incapacity, as exception to informed consent, 146
Incentives. *See* Financial incentives
Individual risk incentives, 171
Industrialization
  of behavioral health care, 131–133
  as opportunity, 139
Industrial Revolution, 131–132
Inflation, 91. *See also* "Health care cost crisis"
Information, and quality care, 245

Informed consent, 143–145
  exceptions to, 145–147
  and managed care, 158–161
Integrated delivery systems
  administrative psychiatry within, 76–79
  and antitrust laws, 206
  in managed behavioral health care, 74–76
  preparation for, 82–83
Integrated treatment, of complex cases, 252–254

Javits, Jacob, 197

Leadership, 50, 53–54, 251–252
Legal regulations. *See* Government regulations
Less-is-more payment method, 12
Liability. *See* Malpractice liability
Lundberg, George, 176–177

Malpractice liability, 195–196
  and ERISA, 199–200
  MCOs' protection from, 218
  of psychiatrists, 50
  UR contractors' protection from, 211
Managed behavioral health care
  collaboration with academic psychiatry, 111–112
  barriers to, 112–115
  objectives for, 115–119
  suggestions for, 119–121
  health care reform and market forces, 72–73
  integrated delivery systems, 74–76
  administrative psychiatry within, 76–79
  preparation for, 82–83
  overview, 71–72
  and public mental health programs, 81–82
  quality management systems, 32–33, 79–81
  See also Medical marketplace
Managed care
  and confidentiality, 161–165
  cost control measures, 12–14
  and informed consent, 158–161
  medicine as product, 242–243
  outcome studies, 243–244
  and physician-patient relationship, 151–158
  and practice of medicine, 149–150
  public backlash against, 99–100
  quality management systems in, 32, 33
  stages of
    capitation, 221–228
    carve ins, 229–231
    selective contracting networks, 214–221
    utilization review, 210–213
  as threat to private practice, 90–96

Managed care *(continued)*
See also Health maintenance organizations; Market discipline paradigm; Medical marketplace; Moral paradigm; Political paradigm; Preferred provider organizations; Professional paradigm
Managed care organizations (MCOs). See Health Maintenance Organizations; Managed care; Preferred provider organizations
"Managed competition," 97
Market discipline paradigm, 187, 190
and capitated systems, 224–228
and ERISA, 196–197
vs. government regulation, 190–193
and oligopsony purchasing power, 203–207
and selective contracting, 216–221
and utilization review, 212–213
Medicaid, 5–6, 195
Medical emergencies, as exception to informed consent, 145–146
"Medically necessary," interpretation of, 193–195
Medical marketplace
challenge of value in, 127–129

emergence of, 15–21
and health care reform, 72–73
private practice in, 100–103
role of psychiatrists in, 42–44
See also Managed behavioral health care; Managed care
Medical model, 240
Medical savings accounts (MSAs), 98
Medical schools
carve ins for, 229–231
carve outs for, 226–228
Medicare, 5–6
and DRGs, 221–222
and PPS, 12
and RBRVS, 11
shift to managed care, 195
Medication management, 251
Medicine, Money, and Morals (Rodwin), 169–170, 177–178
Mental health sites
psychiatrists' role in, 46–48
public, 4–5, 16
Metropolitan Ins. Co. v. Massachusetts, 201
Moral paradigm
focus of, 187
and malpractice lawsuits, 195–196
and managed care, 188–189
Moral responsibility, models of, 142–143. See also Ethical issues
"Moral therapy," 53

Index

More-is-better incentives. *See* Fee-for-service (FFS) reimbursement
Morreim, E. Haavi, 154–156, 157

National Alliance for the Mentally Ill, 188
National Committee for Quality Assurance, HEDIS 3.0, 33
Negative gatekeeping, 172, 173
Negotiated discounts, 209, 214–221

Oligopsony purchasing power, 204–207
of PPOs, 214–215, 216
role of, 203–204
Oregon Plan, 194–195
Organized health care systems. *See* Managed care
Osheroff–Chestnut Lodge debate, 219
Outcomes data
on managed care, 243–244
on private practice, 98–99
Outcomes management, 79–81, 137–138
Outpatient consultation, with PCPs, 65–66
Outpatient practice, in new medical marketplace, 16–17
Outpatient psychiatrists, 89

Paradigms. *See* Market discipline paradigm; Moral paradigm; Political paradigm; Professional paradigm

Patient advocacy, 153, 179
Patient Protection Act, 160–161
Patients
high-risk, management of, 60–61
reactions to new medical marketplace, 17–18
"10 Cs" of quality for, 30
See also Physician-patient relationship; Psychiatrist-patient relationship
Physician-hospital organizations (PHOs), 51–52, 223
Physician organizations (POs), 51–52
Physician-patient relationship, 141–142, 165–166
confidentiality in, 147–148, 161–165
Hippocratic model of, 241–242
informed consent in, 143–147, 158–161
and managed care, 151–158
models of moral responsibility, 142–143
violations of, 99–100
See also Psychiatrist-patient relationship
Physician review organizations (PROs), 149
Physicians, in new medical marketplace, 18–19
Point-of-service options, 97–98
Political paradigm, 187, 189–190, 197

Positive gatekeeping, 172
Practice guidelines, 133–137
  and financial incentives, 180
  and "medically necessary" care, 193
Practice management, 52–53
Preferred provider organizations (PPOs)
  oligopsony purchasing power of, 214–215
  structure of, 150
  See also Managed behavioral health care; Managed care
Primary care physicians (PCPs)
  as gatekeepers, 230
  outpatient consultation with, 65–66
  role in carve-out arrangements, 225
Primary care sites, role of psychiatrists in, 48–49
Privacy, 91
  federal legislation proposal for, 163–164
  in new medical marketplace, 100
  See also Confidentiality; Ethical issues
Privacy Protection Study Commission of 1977, 163
Private practice, 87, 103–104
  diversity of, 89–90
  in new medical marketplace, 100–103
  outcomes data on, 98–99
  strengths of, 88–89

systems vs. individuals, 90–92
  trends
    negative, 92–96
    opposing, 97–98
    positive, 96–97
  See also Solo practice
Productivity-based bonus incentives, 171
Professional determinations, for quality health services, 26–29
Professional paradigm, 187, 188
  interpretations of "medically necessary," 193–195
  and malpractice lawsuits, 195–196
Prospective Payment System (PPS), 12
Psychiatric consultation, 47–48
Psychiatric hospitals. *See* Hospitals; Mental health sites
Psychiatric residents, reimbursement proposal for, 116–118
Psychiatric science
  guidelines and outcomes in, 133–138
  revolution and roots of, 124–127
Psychiatric training. *See* Academic psychiatry
Psychiatrist-patient relationship
  privacy and continuity in, 91–92
  in private practice, 88–89
  See also Physician-patient relationship

Psychiatrists
  in carve-out arrangements, 227
  clinical roles, 57–59
    crisis assessment, 60
    management of high-risk patients, 60–61
    outpatient consultation with PCPs, 65–66
    psychopharmacologic management, 64–65
    roles to avoid, 67–70
    in solo practice, 63–64
    systems-oriented practice, 67
    as team members, 61–63
  as employers, 51–53
  as experts, 45–51
  focus on whole patient, 247–249
  and human economies of scale, 226, 227–228, 230–231
  as leaders, 50, 53–54, 251–252
  in new medical marketplace, 19–20, 42–44
  preparation for new delivery systems, 82–83
  as principal physician, 256–257
  and psychotherapy, 254–256
  reimbursement for, 250 (*see also* Financial incentives)
  research contributions, 249–250
  skills of, 250–254
  training of, 249 (*see also* Academic psychiatry)
Psychiatry
  administrative, 76–79
  biomedical foundations of, 240–242
  future of, 239, 257–260
  See also Academic psychiatry; Managed behavioral health care; Managed care; Private practice; Quality care
Psychiatry departments
  carve ins for, 229–231
  carve outs for, 226–228
  See also Academic psychiatry
Psychopharmacologic management, 64–65
Psychotherapy
  provision of, in new medical marketplace, 20
  psychiatrist-patient relationship in, 88–89
  and psychiatrists' future roles, 254–256
Public mental health programs, 73, 81–82
Public mental health sites, 4–5, 16

Quality, definition of, 29–31
Quality care
  clinical essentials of, 244–246
  financial incentives based on, 179–180
  in health services, 23
    current contexts of, 24–31
    structure of, 31–35

Quality care *(continued)*
  new approach to, 129–131
  and outcomes management, 79–81
  and value, 127–129
Quality management systems, 32–33

Rationing, 27, 28, 34, 194
Reagan Administration
  deregulation of health care, 192–193
  implementation of DRGs, 221–222
"Reasonable expectations" of coverage, 156
Referral networks. *See* Selective contracting
Referral regulations, 207
Regulation. *See* Government regulations
Residents, reimbursement proposal for, 116–118
Resource allocation, conflicts among patients, 152–154
Resource-Based Relative Value System (RBRVS), 11
Risk incentives, 76, 171, 173
Rodwin, M. A., *Medicine, Money, and Morals,* 169–170, 177–178
"Rule of austerity," 164

Salary incentives, 171
Scientific determinations, for quality health services, 26–29
Selective contracting, 214–221

Self-insured ERISA plans, 201, 202
Single-hospital plans, 216
Social reforms, in 1960s, 4–7
Social screening process, 249
Solo practice
  in new medical marketplace, 19
  psychiatrists' role in, 63–64
  See also Private practice
Specialist risk, 171
Standard of medical expertise (SME), 155, 156
Standard of resource use (SRU), 155–156
State mental hospitals. *See* Public mental health sites
Stratified scarcity, 155
Supply-side cost control methods, 10, 11
"Supply side engineering," 52
Systems-oriented practice, 67

Teams, psychiatrists in
  leadership role, 50, 53–54, 251–252
  other roles, 61–63
"10 Cs" of quality, 30
Therapeutic privilege, as exception to informed consent, 146
Time, and quality care, 245–246
Traditional doctor-patient model, 142
Training. *See* Academic psychiatry
Treatment, quality of. *See* Quality care

Utilization review (UR), 149, 209
  and computerized databases, 219–220
  and financial incentives, 180
  fourth-party, 210–213
  and oligopsony purchasing power, 205

Value, in new medical marketplace, 127–129
Varol v. Blue Cross and Blue Shield of Michigan, 160

Vertical integration, 209, 222–224
  carve ins, 229–231
  carve outs, 224–228

Waiver exception, to informed consent, 146–147
Wedgewood, Josiah, 132
Wickline v. State, 159, 195–196, 199
Wilson v. Blue Cross of S. Cal., 196, 199
Withholding incentives, 171